LIVING FOODS FOR OPTIMUM HEALTH

A Highly Effective Program to Remove Toxins and Restore Your Body to Vibrant Health

Brian R. Clement
with Theresa Foy DiGeronimo

PRIMA PUBLISHING

To every person who makes a difference
by moving forward and becoming a shining example.

Library of Congress Cataloging-in-Publication Data

Clement, Brian R.
    Living foods for optimum health : a highly effective
program to remove toxins and restore your body to vibrant health /
Brian R. Clement with Theresa Foy DiGeronimo.
        p.   cm.
    Includes index.
    ISBN 0-7615-0258-0
    1. Vegetarianism.   2. Health.   I. DiGeronimo, Theresa Foy.
II. Title.
RM236.C565   1996
613.2'62—dc20   96-4284
                                                                                    CIP

96 97 98 99 AA 10 9 8 7 6 5 4 3 2 1

Printed in the United States of America

All products mentioned in this book are trademarks of their respective companies.

Medical Disclaimer
The medical and health information in this book are based on the training, experience, and research of the author. Because each person and situation is unique, the reader should check with a qualified health professional before following this program. Therefore, the author and publisher specifically disclaim any liability, loss, or risk, personal or otherwise, which is incurred as a consequence, directly or indirectly, of the use and application of the contents of this book.

How to Order
Single copies may be ordered from Prima Publishing, P.O. Box 1260, Rocklin, CA 95677; telephone (916) 632-4400. Quantity discounts are also available. On your letterhead, include information concerning the intended use of the books and the number of books you wish to purchase.

Contents

6
Becoming a Living-Foods Vegetarian   109

7
Getting the Most from the Hippocrates Health Program   123

8
Shopping For Your Health   143

9
In the Kitchen with Living Foods   163

10
Eating in the Real World   181

11
Time to Eat: Living-Foods Recipes   187

Foreword

by Coretta Scott King

There are many dimensions to a full and successful life, but my half-century in the area of human development and equality has vividly taught me the essential and fundamental need that each of us has to create abundant personal health on whatever road of life we choose.

One can acquire the tools necessary to enjoy a healthful and harmonious existence by creating a healthy body through nutrition and exercise, a healthy mind through positive throught and peace, and a healthy spirit through commitment and faith. These all contribute to a symbiotic humanity that allows all of us the freedom to reach our greatest potential.

There are endless ways we can improve our future, but none is more vital than commitment to a healthful lifestyle. In recent years I have become acquainted with Brian R. Clement of Hippocrates Health Institute and their work that spans several decades. Brian's candid message of taking responsibility for one's life gives each of us who heed the call infinite possibilities through the development of complete health. On this road of challenge and change, harmony and peace prevail in the very places that confusion and anger reigned. One acquires a sense of deeper devotion to God and nature.

There are hundreds of thousands of people worldwide that now embrace the Hippocrates lifestyle. *Living Foods for Optimum Health* is a landmark guide to the essentials of healthy living. There is no doubt in my mind that Brian's book is being presented at the right place and the right time for the whole of humanity. When reading this practical and easy to understand message, open your heart and mind. You will find yourself entering the new millennium with a healthy body, mind, and spirit.

Introduction

Every three weeks the Hippocrates Health Institute in West Palm Beach, Florida, welcomes a new series of guests. Many arrive with a variety of health concerns—from tumors to diabetes, from arthritis to digestive difficulties. Others who visit the institute are healthy and determined to maintain that precious gift. In either case, the Hippocrates Health Program helps them cleanse and detoxify their systems and offers them personal control over their health and well-being.

Twenty-five years ago, the institute drew me like a beacon of light guiding me away from my disconnected and unhealthy lifestyle. The Hippocrates Health Institute had an international reputation in pioneering the "take-personal-responsibility" approach to health and life and I wanted to be a part of this growing field. Since then, I have risen through the ranks to my present position as director and have watched tens of thousands of people from around the world learn how to live better, more productive, and healthier lives by using the information we provide at our Lifestyle Change Center, as well as through the many books, videos, and cassette tapes we distribute worldwide.

My work gets more exciting by the day, and now I'm overjoyed to gather the basics of all this information into this book. The opening chapters support the validity of the Hippocrates Health Program by closely examining the evolution of toxic malnutrition in the twentieth century. You'll follow the emergence of our malnourished society through the fast-paced developments in agricultural technologies, in the proliferation of chemical and pharmaceutical products in the food chain, in consumer expectations, and in government involvement in the food industry. You'll examine the kinds of food that have sat on our kitchen tables throughout the past century and the technological discoveries and social attitudes that made them popular. You'll explore technological breakthroughs such as wheat processing that gave us nonspoiling white bread, food additives that increased the shelf-life of baked goods, and pesticides that protected thousands of acres of crops. You'll also learn how these technologies' positive intents resulted in a negative effect on our health.

In following chapters, you'll take an analytical look at the nutritional myths we've all been raised on. You'll examine those "balanced" meals that combine chemically combustible elements and cause an epidemic of gastrointestinal ailments. You'll uncover the fallacies of popular weight-loss diets and the dangers of good ol' home cooking.

The Hippocrates Health Program uses the mistakes of the twentieth century to point us in a new direction—a direction that uses what we know about the indisputable healing and restorative powers of living foods to bring physical and mental health to the people of the twenty-first century. I've written this book so that you can have a handy, practical, step-by-step guide to living-foods vege-tarianism. This is a way of life that restores harmony to the body through the use of fresh, raw, and living foods that nourish, cleanse, and alkalinize the body by the combined action of their nutritional

components: vitamins, minerals, amino acids, liquids, complex carbohydrates, fiber, and especially oxygen and enzymes. You'll learn how
to shop for living foods and how to prepare them. You'll learn how to
germinate and sprout your own beans and grains. You'll learn how to
"cook" without the heat that destroys oxygen and enzymes. You'll also
learn how to get the most out of your new diet by making lifestyle
changes that include a positive attitude, exercise, colon cleansing,
relaxation, fasting, dry skin brushing, aromatherapy, sauna, steam
baths, whirlpool, massage, and electrical frequency therapy.

At the end of this book, you'll find a collection of my family's
favorite recipes. These will give you a solid foundation for creating
tasty and visually appealing daily meals to help you attain the goal of
the Hippocrates Health Program: To accomplish a mind- and body-
cleansing program that is coupled with a totally toxic-free diet. This
diet allows your body to use its own inner healing mechanisms without interference from external toxins. This book is your guide to living healthy in a polluted and malnourished world. In summoning the
courage of commitment needed to set out in this new direction, you
will gain abundant well-being.

For further information on the Hippocrates Health Institute, please write:

Hippocrates Health Institute
1443 Palmdale Court
West Palm Beach, Florida 33411

Acknowledgments

I want to acknowledge the help and support of my predecessors
Ann Wigmore and Victor Kulvinskas, my wife and codirector
Anna Maria, my children Daly, Danielle, and Gail, my parents, and
my staff at the Hippocrates Health Institute, as well as Theresa.

—B. C.

1

What We Know Now That We Didn't Know Then

What a century! The scientific and technological breakthroughs made in our quest to understand the biological needs of the body have astounded us throughout the 1900s. And the Hippocrates Health Institute has been very much a part of this exciting time. For more than 40 years, people from all around the world have come to the institute to learn more about health and longevity. The institute began in 1957 with the concept that the human body is a self-healing and self-rejuvenating organism if given the proper tools and environment. Founded by Ann Wigmore and Viktoras Kulvinskas, the institute's purpose was to collect and implement research data focusing on the attainment of optimum health through the use of live, enzyme-rich foods that detoxify the body and renew and build all of its cells.

At first considered eccentric, The Hippocrates Health Institute now enjoys renown as a premier health center. We are seeing a dramatic shift in the public's attitude about the role that diet and lifestyle play in our overall health and longevity. More and more people are realizing that in deviating from the natural order, we lose something invaluable and life-giving. Indeed, it is no longer considered "natural" for people to eat a diet that is overcooked, overprocessed, denatured, sprayed, and possibly even irradiated before being preserved and packaged. This shift in attitude has paved the way for this book.

A LOOK BACK

But how did we get to this point? Let's take a quick look back.

More than any other time in history, the past century has experienced a revolution in food manufacturing and consumption that has drastically affected the world's diet and attitude. Before, the average person's knowledge of the relationship between food and health was nebulous at best; it wasn't until just before the First World War that we were even aware of the existence of substances called vitamins. And it was only in the 1920s that Dr. Royal Lee invented supplements. The journey from the time of these discoveries to the present has been packed with many changes—many of them controversial.

At the turn of the century, the primary nutritional concerns were the safety and adulteration of food. A heightened awareness of bacteria led to the establishment of the Food and Drug Administration (FDA), U.S. Department of Agriculture (USDA) inspections, and pasteurization.

Next, we began to demand consistent food quality with stable prices. This demand was closely linked with the expansion in the manufacture and distribution of brand-name goods and advertising. In the 1940s, Dr. Hazel Stiebling and her colleagues at the USDA established the first "Recommended Daily Allowances."

In the 1950s, Americans became enamored with the supermarket. Canned and processed foods, chemical preservatives, and convenience and fast foods became the rage. In 1954, TV dinners made their first appearance and convinced homemakers that fast was best.

In the 1960s, a new food consciousness accompanied social activism. Meat was out for many because it was viewed as a form of cruelty to animals; brown rice was in. At the same time, the medical establishment was beginning to note the link between diet and health. In 1968, the American Heart Association was the first to suggest that Americans limit their intake of fat to about one-third of their total calories.

In 1971, the USDA issued a landmark report on the benefits from human nutrition research. Data showed that poor nutrition was related to all major health problems. The report summarized the estimated magnitude of the potential benefits and savings from nutritional research for these problems. Since 1971, the role of nutrition in health and disease has come under heightened scrutiny.

In the 1980s, the conclusions of long-term research projects such as the Framingham Heart Study were beginning to establish the link between certain foods and risk factors for disease. Nutritionists began drawing up diet plans that would lower the risk of ailments such as heart disease and colon cancer. The National Academy of Sciences, the National Cancer Institute, and the American Cancer Society all began recommending lowfat diets. Phytochemicals (naturally occurring chemicals that help fight cancer and other diseases) were discovered in our foods. People began seriously considering the relationship between what we eat and how we live; the 1980s saw a jury genuinely weigh whether a killer might have been driven to crime by eating too many Twinkie snackcakes.

In the 1990s, the evolutionary process continued. This decade has brought sweeping international changes in the way we categorize and label foods. The FDA's Nutrition Labeling and Education Act of 1990 gave us the most sweeping changes in food labeling in more than twenty years. Manufacturers of all meat, poultry, and processed foods must provide package labels that help consumers gauge their intake of fat, cholesterol, sodium, sugar, vitamins, and fiber. The law also regulates the definitions of "health" terms such as *fat free, low cholesterol, lite,* and *high fiber.*

Also, the four basic food group theory created by the USDA in 1956 (which many of us memorized in school) was replaced in 1992 with a tiered pyramid concept. The traditional food wheel had outlined four food groups—meats, dairy, vegetables/fruits, and grains—but it didn't clarify how to prioritize these building blocks in relationship to daily eating habits. The new pyramid advocates a diet heavy in grains, fruits, and vegetables—with decreasing amounts of milk, yogurt, cheese, meats, nuts, fats, and sweets. This represented a significant departure in how nutrition would be taught henceforward.

VEGETARIAN '90s

In the early 1990s, we saw meat becoming a four-letter word and vegetables moving to the center of the plate. This shift has been a long time coming. Back in 1917, a mass experiment in vegetarianism was conducted with more than three million subjects. In a rationing program in Denmark, the government stopped feeding the nations' grain to livestock in order to provide meat, and instead fed the grain directly to the people. When the death rate was calculated for the year that followed, they found that the overall mortality rate from disease was by far the lowest in their recorded history.[1] More experiments were conducted around the world throughout the twentieth century, and now few can argue the proven relationship between diet and health.

A landmark study, called "Diet, Lifestyle and Mortality in China," was published by Oxford and Cornell University Press in 1990. These researchers set out to determine what humans should be eating. At first they couldn't find a vegetarian population that stayed in one place generation after generation, until they found a group in China that they used as their control group. After studying the diet, lifestyle, and mortality of many groups around the world and comparing it to their control group, the researchers determined that every man, woman, and child on the planet should be vegan-vegetarians.[2]

We've known of these studies, and we've experimented with their results, but instead of learning their lessons we strayed further from the truth. According to a report from the National Academy of Sciences called *Diet and Health,* the average American intake of meat and dairy products has skyrocketed since consumption was first documented in 1909. We consumed nearly three hundred pounds of grain products per person per year at the turn of the century. Today grain consumption has fallen to half that amount. Milk, milk products, and meat consumption has risen 50 percent, and chicken consumption has risen 280 percent.[3] During this century, we have exchanged a plant-based diet for a meat-based diet. The results have proven to be disastrous for our health and the environment. Now on the threshold of a new century, there is evidence that the mainstream population in developed nations is ready to join the majority of the world in embracing vegetarianism as the superior road to good health. (The Disney theme parks now offer vegetable burgers. Surely this is a sign of changing times!)

THE NEXT STEP

It was not a giant step from a lacto-ovo vegetarian diet (which excludes meat, poultry, and fish but includes eggs and dairy products) to the now increasingly popular vegan-vegetarian diet (which excludes all dairy products and eggs). Like meat products, the production of dairy products relies on the suffering and sacrifice of animals. (We've all heard about or have seen the pictures of the thousands of hens crammed into hen houses and cows penned in stalls too small to allow them to even turn around.) On the health front, the cellular damage to the human body caused by ingesting dairy products replicates the damage done by the similarly high-fat, high-cholesterol, and high-protein content of meat.

WHAT WE LOST ALONG THE WAY

For the first time in this century, agreement is unified among prominent food authorities about the value of a vegan-vegetarian diet. The facts are well documented. So why are so many Americans still hooked on meat and dairy diets? The answer is not a secret. Today's nutritional attitudes are dictated by commercial industries that support only what is profitable. Meat and dairy products make big money; vegetables, fruits, grains, seeds, and nuts do not. Dairy and meat proponents claim that vegetarian diets do not supply us with adequate amounts of vitamins, minerals, and protein. They say this even though it is now well known that the role of vitamins, minerals, and proteins in maintaining health was at first misunderstood and is now grossly exaggerated.

But again, this exaggeration is rooted in the profitability of such industry-created measurements. Vitamins, minerals, and proteins are visible, tangible components of health. They can be synthetically created in the laboratory. They can be bottled and sold. And they are indiscriminate in the foods they choose to call home. They are found in meat and dairy products and even in Cheese Doodles and chips. They can be used to "enrich" processed foods. They give the National Dairy Association and the National Livestock and Meat Board a base on which to stand their claims of nourishment—even the ones that are erroneous.

JINGLES SPEAK LOUDER THAN SCIENTIFIC RESEARCH

Now that international interest in the relationship between diet and health has grown, special interest groups bombard us with "medical" information. The news on osteoporosis is a perfect example. We've all heard that to avoid the ravages of osteoporosis women need to increase their intake of calcium by drinking more milk (or the new calcium-fortified juices and antacid tablets!). But osteoporosis is not first a disease of calcium deficiency. It is a disease of excess protein. Animal and dairy products are full of sulfur-rich proteins. Sulfur makes extra acid in the body; as acids wash through the bones, they dissolve calcium, which is then eliminated through the urine. This only happens with animal protein and it has a name: protein-induced hypercalciuria, which simply means too much calcium going out in the urine. There's no doubt that the findings reported by Drs. Lindsay, Oddoye, and Margen in the *American Journal of Clinical Nutrition* are true: "High protein diets cause a negative calcium balance, even in the presence of more than adequate dietary calcium. Osteoporosis would seem to be an inevitable outcome of continued consumption of a high protein diet."[4] Even calcium tablets and daily doses of milk can not keep up with the calcium lost to the excess protein.

Unfortunately, the dairy and meat industries speak louder than medical journals. Their multimillion-dollar advertising campaigns ignore what even the most conservative medical investigators no longer deny—excess protein robs our bones of strength. With their high protein content, milk and meat actually contribute to the accelerating development of osteoporosis. Certainly most people do not know that one teaspoon of sea kelp mixed in a glass of water gives approximately a thousand times more calcium (without animal protein) than an eight-ounce cup of milk. You can bet you won't hear that information pop up in a catchy jingle.

This false fanfare is not new. Remember when the manufacturers of Wonder Bread convinced your family in the 1960s that white bread could build strong bodies in twelve ways? Wonder has since had to recant. But we were duped.

WHAT WE KNOW NOW

At the same time that advertising was turning our heads away from the facts, research into the nutritional needs of the body continued on its silent, persistent way—with outstanding results. We learned that vitamins, minerals, and protein alone can not keep us healthy. We now know, without a doubt, that there are six vital components of good health that can not be gained with a diet that relies on meat, dairy products, and processed or "enriched" foods. These are the following:

1. enzymes
2. a pH-balanced blood supply that is more alkaline than acid

3. oxygenated blood to feed all the body's systems, organs, and brain
4. a healthy system of digestion and elimination
5. an uncompromised immune system
6. electrically charged tissues and cells that have the ability to build strong organs, muscles, and bones

The Hippocrates Health Program that will be outlined in detail in later chapters focuses on a diet and lifestyle that embraces these six requirements of health.

WHAT WE DIDN'T KNOW THEN

We've learned a lot in the twentieth century. As we enter the twenty-first century, we're ready to take the next logical step. It's time to combine the wisdom we gained about our body's needs with what we're now learning about the high-tech food industry. It's time to exclude from our diet all red meat, poultry, fish, dairy, eggs, additives, processed foods, and even fruits and vegetables that have been irradiated or sprayed with pesticides. These recommendations are based on reams of research and the institute's decades of working with tens of thousands of individuals who personally testify to the life-zapping effects of these foods. Consider just these few facts that we didn't know in the first half of this century, but which are proven scientifically today:

Fat Facts

If you were raised on typical school lunches, then you know that you can't leave the table without eating your meat and finishing your milk. But maybe you didn't know then that these mandated meals were a sanctioned prescription for ill health in later years. A diet that includes meat and dairy products wreaks havoc in the body for a variety of reasons. But for a moment let's focus on fat.

When you draw blood from a person and let it sit for an hour or two, you will see the thick, red, clotted blood fall to the bottom of the test tube and the yellowish serum of the blood rise to the top. This is a normal, healthy occurrence. However, the serum of a person who has recently eaten a cheeseburger will be thick and greasy white; it will stick to the sides of the tube like glue. This is the fat from the burger and the butterfat from the cheese. Specialists call the phenomenon lipemia, and it happens every time you eat a fatty meal. The blood stays this way for about four hours until your liver can clear it out of the bloodstream. When you have a cream doughnut for breakfast, a burger for lunch, fried chicken for dinner, and ice cream for a late-night snack, you're keeping your blood fatty all day long. Blood that never gets a chance to clear out the fatty residue for decades is going to stick to the arteries and clog up the blood flow.

Red meat, chicken, and fish are the top sources of fat and cholesterol in the Western diet. The second source is the yolk of hen's eggs. The third source comes from milk. Milk is a high-fat fluid exclusively designed for turning a sixty-five-pound calf into a four hundred-pound cow in the first year. The dairy industry takes this high-fat liquid, skims off the butterfat, and concentrates it into other even higher-fat "foods" such as butter, ice cream, milk chocolate, sour cream, yogurt, cheese. All of these things, eaten year after year, frequently lead to cardiovascular disease—the number one cause of death in our society.

The atherosclerotic material these high-fat foods create clogs arteries all throughout the body. It's just a matter of which artery to which organ clogs up first to give you the symptoms of a specific disease. If the fat builds up in the arteries going to the brain, you will suffer a stroke. If it clogs an artery going to your kidney, you'll suffer kidney failure or high blood pressure. If the fatty material accumulates in the aorta that takes blood from the heart down to the abdomen and legs, the artery walls become damaged and weakened and they lose their strength; the high pressure in the artery causes the blood vessel to balloon out causing an aneurysm, which can then rupture, leading to emergency surgery or death. If the fatty mixture clogs an artery going to the heart, you will suffer chest pain called angina pectoris; if it clogs the blood flow completely, you will have a heart attack. This is all the same disease caused by animal fat and suffered by people who eat animal products. You will never see these diseases in living-food vegetarians.

Dairy Warning

In addition to excess fat, dairy products contain these six substances that can create imbalance and disease within the human body:

- bovine protein
- butterfat
- lactose sugar
- chemical contaminants
- bovine leukemia viruses
- bovine growth hormones

A common reaction to such an assault by a foreign protein in our immune system is an outpouring of mucus from the nasal and throat membranes. The resulting mucus flow can create the chronic running noses, persistent sore throats, hoarseness, bronchitis, and recurring ear infections that plague a high percentage of our children.

A Cow in Every Kitchen

We used to think that we needed red meat for its protein. Now we know that's bull. (Excuse the pun.) As we'll see in later chapters, there are plenty of other foods that give us all the protein we need. What we do get from red meat (in addition to a coronary thrombosis caused by too much fat) are things common sense says you don't want on your shopping list. These include the following:

- excess protein, which can cause tumors, create stones, or contribute to obesity
- indigestible waste that clogs the digestive system

- growth hormones used to fatten cattle—which, when consumed by humans, have been shown to lower the age of menses in young girls and promote impotence in men and change our sexual demeanor
- antibiotics used to ward off common animal infections that leave the animal riddled with antibiotic-resistant bacterial strains that are passed on to us
- E. coli bacteria, which contaminates meat when the cows' feces splatter during slaughter. (The Centers for Disease Control and Prevention estimate that twenty thousand people fall sick each year as a result of E. coli infection, resulting in bloody diarrhea, fever, and stomach cramps. About 7 percent of the infected are hospitalized, and forty to sixty people, mostly children, die.)

In sum, we gain absolutely no nutritional benefit from the fifteen cows the USDA estimates the average American consumes in a lifetime.

Poultry

Some health enthusiasts eat chicken because they think white meat doesn't contain the fat and protein of red meat. This is absolutely false. Poultry is not a lean meat. It contains just as much fat as red meat because the muscle of any animal contains fat. (You can see this for yourself when you watch the fat separate from the meat in your chicken soup.) In addition to fat, it contains the same indigestible waste—and the same problem with hormones, antibiotics, and bacteria—found in red meat.

Fish Findings

Some studies have shown that the omega-3 oil (an essential fatty acid) found in fish reduces the risk of heart disease. Right from the start, I believed this to be based on bogus research. The politics of these studies—paid for by pharmaceutical companies seeking an extremely low cost way to use fish oil that had been previously extracted and thrown away—brings out the skeptic in me. Sure enough, a scientific controversy is now brewing. In 1995, the Harvard School of Public Health published a study in the *New England Journal of Medicine* reporting that eating a lot of fish did not result in a healthier heart.[5] I'm not surprised; we already know that the highest rate of osteoporosis on the planet is found in Eskimo women because of all the fatty fish they eat. The same diet surely cannot reduce the risk of heart disease.

Putting the omega-3 debate aside, the overall problem of fish farming and commercial fishing from our polluted waters gives us all reason to exclude fish from our diet. A variety of bacteria, viruses, parasites, and toxins can plague fish and the people who eat them. Some can be extremely debilitating and even deadly; the Centers for Disease Control and Prevention estimates that Americans suffer at least 325,000 cases of food-borne illnesses from fish annually. Ciguatera poisoning is the most frequently reported seafood-related disease in the United States. Because ciguatoxin is odorless and colorless, it's very difficult to tell if a fish is contaminated. Scombroid poisoning occurs when certain types of fish (most often tuna, bonito, mackerel, and mahimahi) are handled improperly and spoil after being caught. Paralytic shellfish poisoning is caused by a toxic agent found in clams, scallops, and other shellfish. The poison is not destroyed by freezing, salting, or drying, nor by common cooking methods of steaming, baking, or frying. Salmonella, hepatitis A, and various intestinal viruses also infect seafood.

Testing seafood for bacteria is no guarantee of safety because viruses do not show up in these tests. Dr. Kathy Kirkland of Duke University and Dr. Sharon McDonnell of the Centers for Disease Control and Prevention reported on the presence of viruses in cooked oysters at a 1995 infectious-disease conference sponsored by the American Society for Microbiology. The viruses spread through fecal contamination of the shellfish and cause vomiting and other intestinal ills in humans. These viruses are the leading cause of shellfish-associated illness. Because there is no way of telling whether shellfish are infected or not, just how many people get sick from food poisoning is not known. We accept the flu-like symptoms as an unavoidable virus without ever knowing its source.

To test the scope of this problem, the producers of the ABC television program *PrimeTime Live* recently bought fifty pounds of fish from markets in New York, Boston, Chicago, and Baltimore. Then the fish were tested for contamination. Twenty percent had bacterial levels higher than would be safe for humans to eat. About 40 percent contained human fecal matter at a higher level than anyone should consume.[6] Studies from around the world have also found that pesticides from a class of chemicals known as organochlorines have found their way into the food chain—most notably in fish who feed in waters contaminated by industrial and agricultural runoff. An Environmental Protection Agency (EPA) study published in 1992 found DDE, a chemical resulting from the breakdown of the pesticide DDT, in more than 98 percent of 388 mostly freshwater sites. DDT was banned twenty-two years ago, yet it is still appearing in plates of seafood. Several other hazardous chemicals (PCBs and mercury, for example) turned up in more than 90 percent of the site sample.[7] Not only are these toxins tenacious once they enter animal tissues, but they can mimic, amplify, or block natural sex hormones such as estrogen and testosterone. This, many believe, explains why the rates of breast and testicular cancer have soared in humans, and why male sperm counts in the industrialized world have plummeted by a startling 50 percent since the dawn of the "chemical revolution" that began after the Second World War. In addition, developmental psychologists Joseph and Sandra Jacobson at Wayne State University in Michigan have conducted studies finding that children born of mothers who had regularly eaten contaminated fish weighed less than average at birth, had smaller heads, and as they matured, began to show decreases in short-term memory and attention span.[8]

Along with bacterial poisons and environmental toxins, fish certainly contains the same artery clogging fat as meat and poultry. And as an added detraction, we know that fish carry more parasites and amoebas than any other source.

Additives

Food additives have served many purposes over the years. In the early nineteenth century, wholesalers and retailers looked for ways to increase the quantity and reduce the price of scarce foods. They often did this by bulking up the genuine article with a cheap additive. Pepper, for example, was often adulterated with a commodity known as "pepper dust," which appears to have consisted of the sweepings from the storeroom floor. Cocoa powder often contained a large percentage of brick dust.

Additives were also used to achieve visual appeal. The rainbow hues of sweets and candies were produced by the highly poisonous salts of copper and lead. Most commercial bread was loaded with alum. And it's an interesting fact that Gloucester cheese frequently acquired its rich orange color from additions of red lead.

Today our food supply is largely protected from these kinds of additives. But in their place, a wide variety of nonfood and processed-food materials—never imagined at the beginning of the century—have crept into the food chain. We routinely consume residues of radioactivity, mercury, and organochloride pesticides. The government assures us that each separately is a negligible threat (as is brick dust). But what about the total sum of additives one consumes on a daily diet of processed foods? The EPA acknowledges that there has been no way for researchers to measure cumulative effects. What we do know is that there is a measured amount of pesticides that one can absorb without ill effect in an average seventy-five year lifespan. We also know that in North America, most one-year-old babies have acquired this seventy-year maximum.[9]

Processed Foods

Beginning about 1950, foods containing legal chemical additives became increasingly prevalent as highly processed foods became a predominant portion of the diet. Today, the average American consumes 150 pounds of processed food additives each year. This is not an astounding statistic considering that during this last century more than three thousand different additives have found their way into our food. Why so many? Four common reasons are given for including artificial substances in processed foods:

1. Manufacturers use "taste improvers" to restore flavor lost from canning, drying, and freezing.
2. Additives maintain the visual appeal of many prepacked foods until consumption.
3. To appease weight-conscious consumers, traditional ingredients are replaced by "non-fattening" ones.
4. Many food products are "vitamin-enriched" with synthetic nutrients.

A warning: Recent long-term studies are showing that the toxic by-products and wastes from these chemical-laden foods accumulate in the body, causing cell mutation and eventual cancer.

Irradiation Madness

What happens to living cells when they're irradiated? This sounds like a rhetorical question—of course, they're killed, and their bioelectric field is destroyed. Well, why would we eat food (even "fresh" fruits and vegetables) that have been irradiated? Another rhetorical question. Yet, in many nations irradiation of food to control insects and bacteria and to retard spoilage is widely used.

Fresh fruits and vegetables, fish, poultry, pork, wheat, and herbs are legally irradiated with cesium-137 (a highly radioactive material with a half-life of 30.2 years and a hazardous life span of 600 years). Red meat and seafood are on the waiting list. But are irradiated foods safe to eat? The government's official answer is yes. But scientists from the FDA have acknowledged that irradiation may kill harmless bacteria as well. Harmless bacteria compete with dangerous pathogens, protecting against their reproduction. By killing bacteria with low-dose radiation, we may be establishing a milieu where only the virulent and more dangerous pathogens survive. There's also a question about what the Department of Health and Human Services defines as "low-level" radiation. The 100,000 rads used to kill insects and other organisms on produce amounts to the equivalent of more than three million chest x-rays. No doubt, further research will find this method of food production a big mistake.

Pesticide Perspective

In our own backyards, we wouldn't take a garden fruit or vegetable, spray it with bug spray and then hand it to our children to eat. Yet, increasingly, that's exactly what we do each day with our store-bought produce. Agricultural pesticide use continues to rise (up 170 percent in the last eighteen years). In a survey taken in 1993 and released in 1995, the USDA found residues of 10,329 chemicals on the 7,328 samples tested. Apples had the highest pesticide findings, with 97 percent of those sampled having at least one residue.[10]

Parallel to the increased use of pesticides is the increase in the cancer rate, which now affects one in three Americans. Research has shown a correlation between exposure to some pesticides and the likelihood of getting cancer—one more, very convincing, reason to beware of chemically laden foods. (Be sure to read the information on pesticide-free, organically grown foods in chapter 8.)

Genetically Engineered Foods

Genetic engineering is the latest food manufacturing craze, but it is not new. Back in the 1950s when standardization became the rage, blunt-end carrots were bred so they wouldn't puncture the bag; tomatoes were grown not for taste but for a standard weight precisely divisible into a pound (for example, eight tomatoes to the pound); and even the development of miniature India-rubber mushrooms with nothing to recommend them but their looks became quite popular. Today's sophisticated technology has simply expanded the possibilities—sometimes beyond the borders of sound nutrition.

With the same good and honest intentions that gave us white bread and artificial sweeteners, technology now is able to give us plants that resist insect infestation, frost, and drought; cows with increased milk production; tomatoes that can sit on our counter for two months without rotting; and meat with less fat. In all food groups, genetically manipulated foods are ready for our table. But are we ready for the potential side effects?

Despite the promise of genetically engineered food, very serious problems need to be addressed. This growing field can be used for both good and bad. For good, we may be able to increase crop yields in starving countries. For bad, the manipulation of a nutrient's DNA may have serious, long-term effects on the human body.

We know nutrients have an effect on the chromosomes of the body, so manipulated nutrients might well have a very subtle, but definite, negative impact on our overall health. Genetic engineering alters the chemistry of food by genetically manipulating and combining the DNA of several types of foods. Certainly, this leaves the final product with an unharmonized mineral structure. The question is, Does this arrangement create the potential for mutant nutrients? I believe it does.

Combining DNA from different foods is like taking three people from different countries, putting them together in a small room, and expecting that—because they are all people—they'll understand each other just fine. Similarly, nutrients and minerals can't be extracted from their source and just thrown together. They too need to be able to communicate with each other to be successfully used by the body.

Also of concern is the fact that we don't yet know how DNA alterations affect the electromagnetic charges of living foods that are needed to attract that food to the body's cells for perfect absorption. Like a string of holiday lights that goes out because one bulb is removed, the relationship between nutrients and the body's cells may cease to function if one part of its structure is removed or manipulated. Even though the final product looks like a food, we don't know yet if the nutrient composition is the same harmonious collection that nature created to nurture body cells.

This is all yet to be tested and proven, but we already have evidence of the insidious dangers of genetically engineered foods. Who would have thought that the manipulation of fruit genes could create a final product that is unhealthy? Yet that's what has happened with hybrid apples. Red delicious apples, for example, have fifty times more sugar than their origin apple. Gene manipulation has turned what was a perfect food into a food with excess fructose, which when eaten contributes to a perfect environment for disease. Some people feel the uniform appearance of these apples is worth the trade-off. I disagree.

With this sugar change having been tested and proven, researchers now need to examine the genetically engineered changes in components such as amino acids, which when mutated rob minerals from the bones. We need to know more about the long-term effects of DNA manipulation that transfers fish genes into tomatoes to prolong shelf life, that puts human genes into pork to improve stability and size, that injects synthetic steroids into cattle to enlarge the gene pool. All these technological "advances" have a domino effect that I believe will seriously affect the health of the human body in years to come.

THE RESULT

The results of the relentless, daily assault on the body by highly processed and genetically engineered foods create great tragedies in the so-called civilized world: malnutrition and the eventual breakdown of our immune system, our metabolic processes, and our glandular functions. All the synthetic vitamins and minerals in the world can not save the body from this onslaught. And so, by the hundreds of thousands, we die early deaths each year.

HEALTHY CELLS = LONGEVITY

Why do the life-giving cells of the body degenerate, mutate, and die? Because they are not fed properly. This may sound too simplistic an answer to the question of life and death, but it's fact. The hope of longevity lies in the health of our cells.

The Hippocrates Health Program is not a bandage. It is not intended as a quick fix or a symptom silencer. It is a biochemical approach to health that regenerates the cellular structure of the body. This approach works because the cells of the body are constantly renewing themselves. For example, skin cells take only twenty-eight days to completely regenerate; the heart cells, thirty days; the lungs, seventy days. How logical then, to nurture health through these microscopic and constantly regenerating cells that have the ability to begin anew. That's why the body needs living foods. Unlike cooked, processed, or animal foods, living foods can supply the cells with what they need to grow. Alone, they determine the health and vitality of the cells, and the health of the cells determines the quality of life.

THE ROOTS OF WELLNESS

The twentieth century certainly has not been kind to the cells of mainstream food consumers. After accepting this fact, we need to make a mental shift to find the roots of wellness in a different place—in a living-foods diet. Not only do living foods give our body's cells the vitamins, minerals, and proteins they need, but they also supply the oxygen, enzymes, alkalinity, and bioelectrical charges so vital to cellular health that no other foods offer.

2

The Facts About Living Foods

A diet of living foods is not a new idea. Many ancient cultures knew the value of eating uncooked vegetables and fruits and of germinating and sprouting grains, seeds, legumes, and nuts. In the early 1900s, Dr. Szekely translated the *Essene Gospel of Peace, Books I–IV,* which revealed that the use of live foods in the treatment of disease had been part of the Western and Judaic-Christian tradition for more than two thousand years.[1] The Essenes, a Jewish sect dating from two hundred to three hundred years before the time of Jesus, were said to eat primarily live foods and were reported by anthropological historians to live an average of 120 years.

The curative powers of living foods have long been known to Asian medicine as well. In fact, the use of sprouted seeds for food and medicine is more than twice as old as the Great Wall of China and was even noted in their historical records.

Even in more modern times, the value of a living-foods diet has been gaining scientific support in the medical community for the last one hundred years. In the early 1900s, Dr. Max Gerson discovered the power of living foods for healing his own migraines, and then later for the supposedly incurable disease lupus. He then applied the diet to various diseases, from clogged arteries to mental disorders. Dr. Gerson recognized living foods as a way to rebuild the vital regenerative force of the total organism. In 1928, he used this diet to heal Albert Schweitzer's wife of tuberculosis. Later, he put Schweitzer himself on a living-foods diet to treat his diabetes. As a result, Schweitzer was able to stop using insulin. Dr. Gerson's later work found that living foods improved cellular respiration as well as strengthening the immune system. He began using the diet to treat cancer with great success. His work was highlighted in the extensively documented book, *A Cancer Therapy.*[2]

At the same time, others in the medical and scientific communities were also proving the curative powers of living foods. Works such as "The Influence of Food Cooking on the Blood Formula of Man," presented by Paul Kouchakoff, M.D., at the First International Congress of Microbiology in Paris in 1930,[3] and Dr. Edward Howell's 1946 book, *Food Enzymes for Health and Longevity*[4] brought living foods to the forefront of nutritional studies.

Many others soon began exploring the healing power of living foods. The Danish physician, Kristine Nolfi, switched to living foods to cure her breast cancer. Based on her own positive experiences and her patients', she started the successful Humlegaarden Sanitarium in Denmark. Among the American pioneers of living foods are Paul Bragg, who opened the first health food store in the United States and, of course, Ann Wigmore and her predecessor, Viktoras Kulvinskas, who decades ago founded the Hippocrates Institute—where the curative and restorative powers of living foods were (and still are) sampled first-hand by those who come as guests.

Unfortunately, by the 1950s, the population had become enamored with the supermarket and its canned and processed foods, the promise of chemical preservatives and pesticides, and the lure of fast foods. The value of a living-foods diet was lost in this clamor for convenience. But now, after decades of declining health and rapid aging, the promise of living foods is once again gaining international attention.

NO COOKING TONIGHT!

As we learned in chapter 1, in addition to an adequate daily intake of certain nutrients, a healthy body requires enzymes, pH balance, oxygenated blood, an efficient system of digestion, an uncompromised immune system, and bioactive electrically charged tissues and cells. Let's take a look at the facts that explain why only living foods give the body all these essential food components.

YOU ARE WHAT YOU EAT

The highest quality foods are the natural, living foods. Amino acids are in their finest form, and minerals, vitamins, carbohydrates, trace elements, oxygen, enzymes, and hormones are all present.

Wheatgrass, for example, (a staple of the Hippocrates diet) is largely chlorophyll and contains all the essential amino acids; it is a rich source of vitamins A and D, and is exceptionally high in B vitamins. It is also rich in calcium, phosphorus, iron, potassium, sulfur, sodium, cobalt, and zinc. Wheatgrass juice, together with organically grown, living, fresh produce is the naturally enriched nourishment our bodies were created to enjoy.

Although lots of the foods on the typical dinner table contain the nutrients needed for good health, our habit of cooking these foods destroys their potential. Vitamins, for instance, have an identifiable molecular structure. Because cooking by its very nature is the alteration of molecular structure, a rock-hard potato becomes soft after cooking. In changing the molecular structure, doesn't it make sense that the molecular structure of the vitamins in the food will also change? Of course it does, and the change is most often detrimental to our health.

THE ENZYME ACCOUNT

Enzymes are particularly sensitive to the molecular destruction of cooking. Unfortunately, each of us is given only a limited supply of enzyme energy at birth that must work to keep every body system in working order throughout our lifetime. The only other backup source we have comes from the food we eat—but food cooked above 118 degrees F. kills enzymes! So what happens if you make some big enzyme withdrawals when you catch a virus, do something physically strenuous, face an emotional crisis, breathe unclean air, get extremely angry, and then eat cooked and processed foods? The balance in your enzyme account drops low, is not replenished, and your body faces enzyme bankruptcy.

When this happens, the body puts out an emergency call to enzymes throughout the body. The body will rob enzymes from glands, muscles, nerves, and blood to help in the demanding digestive process. Eventually there is a deficiency of enzymes in those areas, and this, many scientists throughout the world believe, is the real cause of various allergies and diseases. According to medical research compiled by the pioneering enzymologist Dr. Edward Howell, enzyme shortages are commonly seen in a number of chronic illnesses such as allergies, skin disorders, obesity, and heart disease, as well as in aging and certain types of cancer.[5]

The healing power of enzymes is absolute and proven. Almost every regulatory system in our body depends on enzymes and suffers by their depletion: coagulation, inflammation, wound healing, and tissue regeneration, to name just a few. The enzyme account through-out the body is replenished by the living foods we eat as the enzymes are absorbed into the blood to reestablish normal blood-serum enzyme levels. To track the whole-body value of an enzyme-rich diet, researchers have tagged enzyme supplements with radioactive dye and traced them through the digestive tract. They discovered that the tagged enzymes could be found in the liver, spleen, kidneys, heart, lungs, duodenum, and urine.

The Hippocrates diet stops unnecessary waste of enzyme energy and makes daily deposits into the enzyme account. Few withdrawals and large deposits are the key to becoming richly supplied with the metabolic enzymes that are responsible for building, cleansing, and healing the body.

THE BALANCING ACT

Scientists have established a pH (**p**otential **H**ydrogen) scale for measuring the acid/alkaline balance of substances. On this scale, a healthy body is about 30 percent acid and 70 percent alkaline. But typically, the average acid-based diet of meat, cheese, white bread, processed and cooked foods, caffeine, nicotine, and alcohol reverses this proportion, creating a highly acid state and drastically affecting all the body's systems and their ability to function.

To imagine the impact of too much acid in the body, think of the calcifications that form on your car battery. This is exactly what you would see if you photographed the digestive, nervous, or circulatory system in a body that has excess acid smothering the cells necessary for survival. In this state, the cells can not adequately take in nutrients and oxygen and they can not efficiently expel toxins. As the cells suffocate, the body becomes open to disease. In fact, I've never seen a person in a disease state who is not highly acidic.

The reason cooked and processed foods cause acidity in the body is that they lack the oxygen and enzymes necessary for food absorption. As soon as food is heated above 118 degrees F., these elements are wiped out. When a food is not totally digested and absorbed, it's allowed to float around as waste products in the blood stream increasing the acidity level of the body.

This increase in body acid and waste causes a variety of health problems. A 1994 study conducted by the University of California that was published in the *New England Journal of Medicine,* shows a definitive relationship between high body acid and osteoporosis.[6] The researchers found that when post-menopausal women are given a

high-protein diet with lots of meat, their blood became acidic. To
neutralize the acidity, their bones released significant amounts of
calcium and phosphorous, causing a depletion of these minerals.

Even the sensation of pain is sensitive to the level of acidity in
the body. Many who are in chronic pain have acidic accumulations
throughout the nervous system. This excess acid aggravates pain in
the same way you would aggravate a toothache by sticking a pin into
the decaying tooth. The only way to reduce this pain permanently is
to reduce the acid.

Is your pH level properly balanced? A physician or a health-care
professional can test your pH level, or you can do it yourself using
litmus paper available from any pharmacy. It's easy to do once you
understand the basics of pH balance:

The pH scale ranges from the most acidic value of 0 to the most
alkaline value of 14, and compares the number of alkaline-forming
hydroxyl ions (OH^-) to the number of acid-forming hydrogen ions
(H^+). Pure water (H_2O) is made up of one hydroxyl and one hydrogen ion and has a neutral pH of 7. Our bodies, being mostly water,
have an overall pH registering close to 7, with each organ having a
slightly different pH. As cellular functions become overburdened and
acid-forming toxins collect in the cytoplasm, the pH drops. It's believed that a slightly alkaline pH (7.1–7.45) of the cellular structure
results in optimum health; most people of "average" health have a
slightly acid pH (6.5–6.8).

So, give it a try—test your pH level. Most practitioners who use
pH as a reference for overall body chemistry agree that in a healthy
body, both urine and saliva should register *on average* around a pH of
6.5. This reflects a slightly alkaline chemistry (7.1–7.45) in the cytoplasm of cells throughout the body.

Once you know your pH level, the challenge becomes one of
maintaining or regaining the alkalinity in the cytoplasm of the cells. If
you follow the guidelines of the Hippocrates diet, you will get alkalinity from oxygen, enzymes, and the bioactive vitamins and minerals,
with a minimum of waste products that burden the body with acidity.

THE CRY FOR OXYGEN

You know that all life requires oxygen, but you may not know that the foods we eat can rob that life-giving oxygen from our cells, causing disease and death. That's why it's important to be sure that we select foods that feed, rather than rob, oxygen. But how can we know which foods give and which foods take oxygen?

If you recall your early science lesson about photosynthesis, you'll remember that all plants, terrestrial and aquatic, absorb water and carbon dioxide and then give off oxygen as a waste product. That's why botanical food is composed of oxygen in the molecular structure of its chlorophyll content. Chlorophyll is the "blood" of a plant. It is the protein in plant life that gives it its distinctive green or purple color. When compared to a molecule of hemoglobin (the oxygen carrier in human blood) chlorophyll is almost identical. Have you ever thought about what happens to that oxygen when we eat those foods in their living state? It feeds oxygen to our body—the oxygen we need to stay alive and healthy. Only living foods bring that oxygen into the body.

The value of chlorophyll isn't a new discovery. In the early part of the twentieth century, chlorophyll was regarded as a top-notch weapon in the arsenal of pharmacopoeia. Many physicians used it as a treatment for various complaints such as ulcers and skin disease, and as a pain reliever and breath freshener. One report by Dr. Benjamin Gurskin, then director of experimental pathology at Temple University, was published in the *American Journal of Surgery*. Dr. Gurskin discussed more than one thousand cases in which various disorders were treated with chlorophyll. Commenting on his associates' experiences with chlorophyll, he wrote, "It is interesting to note that there is not a single case recorded in which either improvement or cure has not taken place."[7] Later in 1941, *Reader's Digest* published an article called "The Green Magic of Chlorophyll," which discussed the tremendous potential of chlorophyll as a food and medicine.[8]

In the mid-1940s, however, the use of chlorophyll as medicine had reached its peak. Unfortunately, liquid chlorophyll turned out to be highly unstable; it could not be bottled and stored for more than a few hours. A synthetic chlorophyll extract, which was produced by fermenting fresh chlorophyll and bonding it with certain mineral elements proved to be inconsistent and at times caused negative side effects. Chlorophyll as a treatment was then abandoned by the medical profession, despite the dramatic effects indicated in various studies. Chlorophyll and many other natural antiseptics were replaced by faster-acting antibiotics and chemical antiseptics.

Today, the importance of chlorophyll is receiving a great deal of renewed interest. One of chlorophyll's more important functions in the Hippocrates diet is oxygenation of the bloodstream. On a high-fat and high-protein diet, our oxygen supply is greatly reduced. Dr. John Gainer, reporting in the August 1971 issue of *Science News,* stated that even a moderate increase in blood-plasma protein can reduce oxygen levels of the blood by as much as 60 percent.[9] I have found that without sufficient oxygen in our blood, we develop symptoms of low energy, and sluggish digestion and metabolism. These outward signs are harbingers of serious illness to follow.

Deprived of an adequate supply of oxygen, the body becomes ripe for disease. Indeed, in his book, *The Cause and Prevention of Cancer,* Dr. Otto Warburg, winner of a Nobel prize for physiology and medicine, concluded that oxygen deprivation was a major cause of cancer and that with a steady supply of oxygen to all the cells, cancer could be prevented indefinitely.

If oxygen is so important to good health, why are so many of us oxygen-deprived? The automatic act of breathing brings in some oxygen every day, but in our polluted cities and with inactive lifestyles that do not force heavy breathing, most people do not get enough oxygen to power a healthy body. In addition, poor diet compounds the problem. Processed foods contain no oxygen, but even oxygen-rich foods lose their oxygen content when cooked. The aroma of food as it cooks is physical evidence that oxygen molecules are leaving the food. A living-foods diet, on the other hand, offers the body a continual and abundant supply of oxygen.

You'll find many chlorophyll-rich foods on the Hippocrates diet including dark-green leafy vegetables, broccoli, cauliflower, cabbage, and sprouts. To a lesser degree, you can also obtain oxygen from root vegetables, grains, and fruit.

HEALTHY DIGESTION

A healthy body is dependent upon a healthy digestive system. You can't have one without the other. Unfortunately, most doctors concur that the majority of us have colons that cannot efficiently do the job of eliminating toxic waste from the body, leaving us open to chronic and terminal diseases.

Let's take a look at how a healthy colon nurtured with living foods works:

1. The enzymes naturally present in living foods digest the nutrients and break them down into chemical substances so small that they can pass through cells lining the digestive tract and enter the blood stream (contrary to the myth that raw foods are difficult to digest!).
2. The digested fiber-rich foods enter the colon where the nutrients are absorbed by the colon wall and distributed to the body's cells through the bloodstream.
3. The toxic waste from the foods is bound for swift elimination by the friendly lactobacillus family of bacteria present in the colon.
4. The remaining fiber helps to dilute, bind, and deactivate many carcinogens.
5. Waste is eliminated from the body through daily bowel movements.
6. At the same time, the ten trillion cells of the body discharge their own waste into the blood stream, which delivers the toxins to the colon for rapid removal from the body.

Our body's waste products are intended to flow swiftly through a healthy colon like the one in this picture.

Figure 2-1 A healthy bowel.

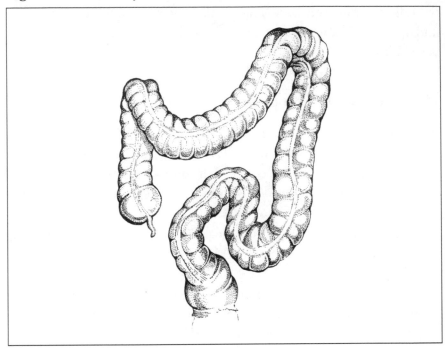

Now consider the process of elimination through a colon stuffed with cooked and processed foods, and meat and dairy products:

1. Foods without enzymes (like cooked vegetables, white bread, pizza, cakes, eggs, milk, meat, and chicken) enter the digestive system, but can not be fully broken down for absorption of nutrients.
2. Without fiber to sweep the remaining toxic waste through the colon, these foods sit in the large intestine. As the colon wall absorbs more and more water, the stools become hard and difficult to eliminate.
3. While sitting in the digestive tract, fats turn rancid, carbohydrates ferment, and protein foods putrefy. This throws poisons back into the body, causing gas, constipation, halitosis, heartburn, headaches, eye troubles, and many other serious conditions.

4. The colon wall begins to absorb the toxins and releases them into the bloodstream as free radicals, or unstable, destructive electrons, that then roam the body seeking healthy cells to invade.

5. As the colon backs up and becomes clogged, the blood can't deposit the waste it picked up from the body's cells. Now overloaded with debris, it can't take any more from the cells. Soon the cells, burdened by their own waste, weaken, mutate, and become open to disease.

6. Even after a bowel movement, some undigested food begins to collect on the walls of the large intestine and disrupts the vital digestive processes of absorption and elimination.

7. Toxic waste pervades the colon because the lactobacillus bacteria that would normally clean up the remains has been destroyed. The antibiotics we consume to fight infection, along with the antibiotics-laden dairy and meat products we eat, kill the healthy bacteria needed to keep the colon healthy.

8. Eventually, the lack of healthy bacteria, combined with the stress from enzyme and fiber deficiency, can cause the colon to lose its strength, shape, and ability to function properly.

Figure 2–2 is a bowel characteristic of what we find in those who eat meats, starches, and cooked foods.

What all this indicates is that the human colon was never meant to handle the digestion of today's typical human diet. The biological evidence shows that humans are herbivorous beings.

Animals who instinctively seek a meat diet have a digestive system to handle the job. The jaw joints of these animals have an up-and-down vertical hinge, and their teeth are overlapping, shearing fangs made for tearing flesh. By contrast, herbivores such as horses and humans have a sliding jaw joint and flat, grinding back molars that allow them to chew in a rotary motion for grinding grains and greens. The stomach acid of carnivorous animals is twenty times that of herbivores because the digestion of flesh requires a lot of acid. If a

Figure 2-2 A diseased bowel.

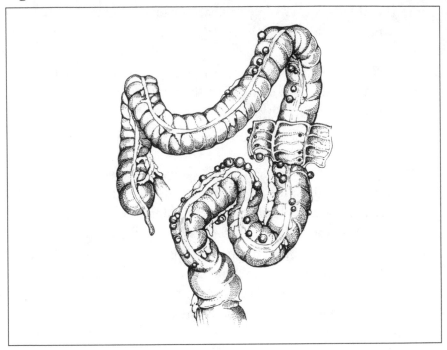

herbivore (like you or me) eats flesh, the body must drastically increase its acid production, which upsets the natural pH balance necessary to maintain health. Carnivorous animals have colons that are constructed to guarantee quick elimination. The bowel of a carnivore is smooth, and it takes waste through a relatively short, straight route of elimination.

As we've seen in earlier illustrations, the bowel of humans, in contrast, is full of pouches and indentations. It follows a long, winding path full of sharp turns. Fatty, processed, and cooked foods cannot pass through this route easily or quickly. (Only living foods, full of digestive enzymes and fiber can move quickly through this maze.) The end result of today's average diet is a grim but indisputable statistic: The greater the intake of cooked and processed foods and animal products, the greater the occurrence of disease.

Figure 2-3 Intestinal system of a carnivore.

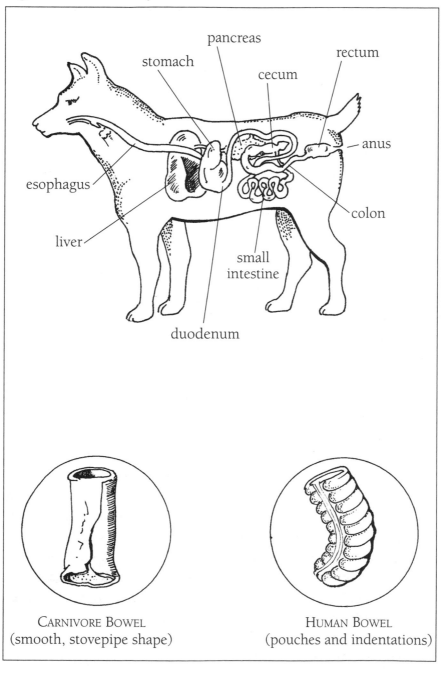

pancreas

stomach

cecum

rectum

esophagus

anus

liver

colon

small
intestine

duodenum

CARNIVORE BOWEL
(smooth, stovepipe shape)

HUMAN BOWEL
(pouches and indentations)

Before true health or reversal of symptoms can occur, waste products must be cleared from the cells, the blood, and the colon. A diet of living foods can do this.

FIGHT BACK

The immune system is one of the most incredible and complex features of our amazing body. When functioning properly, this system of more than two trillion defenders is capable of identifying and eliminating alien invaders while recognizing and then leaving alone our own cells to conduct their business. Whenever we're talking about physiological health, we must consider the immune system because, on an anatomical level, this system is the very reason a person is either healthy or ill.

It is undisputed within the scientific community that when bacteria, or chemicals, or pollen, or any foreign substance enters the body, the immune system's fighter cells (along with numerous other cells) notice the foreign substance and call in the white blood cells. These cells work to destroy and eliminate the intruder.

Now new attention is being given to a 1930 study by Paul Kouchakoff, M.D., that uncovered another important, but lesser known, fact of science. Kouchakoff found that every time we eat cooked foods, we increase the number of white blood cells in our blood stream[10]; the immune system was called upon to protect us! Later in 1943, Otto Warburg further supported Kouchakoff's findings in his study on a process called leukocytosis, which he found occurs when you take a food into the body that has been heated above 194 degrees (a temperature below the boiling point). Leukocytosis causes the food to be recognized as a foreign substance by the immune system and provokes an attack of the fighter white blood cells.[11] This process also occurs when additives, pesticides, and chemically-based supplements enter the body.

Not only are we not getting the oxygen, enzymes, and nutrients from cooked and processed foods, but very importantly, we are also compromising the vitality of the immune system by causing it to work so steadily to destroy and eliminate the food we eat. It's clear that diseases including cancer and AIDS are flourishing because we waste the strength of our immune system fighting cooked, processed, and chemical-laden foods.

BIOELECTRICAL CHARGES

All human tissues and cells are electrically charged; in fact, they work very much like an alkaline battery. Just as an alkaline battery has a positive and a negative pole, a cell has a nucleus and cytoplasm. By the design of nature, the nucleus and cytoplasm of a cell attract opposite charges; the nucleus is the positive "pole" and the cytoplasm is the negative "pole." As the opposite charges collect in their respective areas, the potential for energy flow in a cell increases. The greater the energy potential, the healthier the cell.

Both an alkaline battery and a human cell rely on chemistry to create these opposite charges: certain minerals are negatively charged (alkaline) and another set of minerals are positively charged (acidic). In the human body, these minerals are released during the production of energy (burning of carbohydrates). In addition, light acidic waste by-products are produced. Healthy cells have adequate reserves of negative (alkaline) and positive (acid) charges in their cytoplasms and nuclei, respectively. A living-foods diet replenishes the necessary bioactive alkaline and acid elements to keep cellular energy high and acid waste products low.

Cells in a state of unhealthy decline typically have inadequate reserves of bioactive acids available to the nucleus. More important, there are not enough bioactive alkaline reserves available in the cytoplasm, but there are excess waste acids from various sources accumulating in the cytoplasm. As a result, the charge between the nucleus and cytoplasm decreases and cellular energy resources diminish, allowing further metabolic acids to accumulate. The decreased cellular energy leads to a cycle that results in physical disease. How? The strength and vitality of the electrical fields indicate the strength of the cells. In the human body, the proper electrical charges in and between cells allow the cells to rid themselves of toxins and selectively bring in the appropriate nutrients and oxygen supplies. This process is key to health and longevity. Cells die when the chemistry of the cytoplasm turns acidic and the potential energy drops below a threshold to support this give-and-take life function in the cells. A drop in the electrical potential of the cells is the first step in the disease process. This happens even before laboratory and diagnostic tests can find anything wrong.

The discoverer of a living-foods diet's microelectrical benefits was Professor Hans Eppinger, chief medical doctor at the First Medical Clinic of the University of Vienna. He found that a living-foods diet increased selective capacity of the cells by increasing the electrical potential between the tissue cells and the capillary cells. Dr. Eppinger showed that living foods significantly improved the intra/extra-cellular excretion of toxins and absorption of nutrients. Dr. Eppinger and his colleagues found that living foods were the only kind of food that could restore the microelectrical potential of the tissues once their electrical potential was weakened and the subtle cellular degeneration had begun.

It is believed that living foods get their electrical charges from the highly charged electrons sent to us by the sun. The foods condense the sunlight energy and feed it to our body's cells. Researchers in this field believe that this condensed electrical energy has the ability to awaken relatively inert molecules in our system by either taking an electron or giving them one. That's why the high electrical potential of living foods is an important factor in their healing power.

Dr. Valerie V. Hunt of the Bioenergy Fields Foundation in California has carefully documented her findings about the bio-electricity of cells through Kirlian photography. This is an ultraviolet film technique that exposes the electrical output of any life form. In vivid color, she revealed the changing electroluminescent fields that surround living foods (see Figure 2-4), and the lack of any electrical

Figure 2-4 Kirlian Photography showing the energy field of a sunflower green.

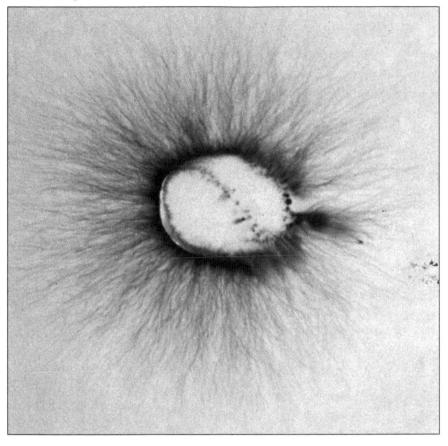

life around junk foods. Kirlian photography studies have also shown the loss of the electrical field in cooked vegetarian foods.[12]

Consider wheat. Depending on how it is prepared, wheat can be an electrically charged or electrically dead. As a living food, it can be sprouted and eaten as is, or ground up and made into an "uncooked" bread or put on a tray and grown into a grass. In these forms, the wheat maintains its electrical charge and an oxygen content that allows a normal bioactive cycle of electrical attraction and assimilation to occur between the nutrient and the human cell when consumed.

The human cell is attracted to the living food as it enters the body with an electrical charge. This allows for thorough absorption of the food's nutrients.

When you take that same piece of wheat, grind it up, cook it, or bake it in a bread, you've destroyed the electrical charge. When that happens, the wheat becomes a renegade as it enters the body; it is not attractive to the cells that need oxygen and enzymes for sustenance, and so it is not able to be wholly absorbed as a nutrient. It is free to roam the body and settle as deposits that suffocate cells, letting them neither take in nutrients nor expel their toxins. For many years, the body will do its best to handle this unrelenting abuse. But over time, it's guaranteed to lose the fight and fall into a diseased state.

Science today can not determine why the body ages and dies, but there's no doubt the answer will come as we more fully examine the individual microscopic cells that become depleted of their electrical charges. We'll also learn that only living foods restore the electrical potential of the body's cells. Only living foods rejuvenate life within the body.

ANTIOXIDANTS

More than fifteen hundred antioxidants have been identified in the foods we eat. These naturally occurring substances combat free radicals that, left unchecked, damage living cells and contribute to a long list of conditions and ailments, including premature aging, heart disease, immunodeficiency, arthritis, cancer, cataracts, allergies, and diabetes. Surely it's no surprise that these disease busters are most abundant and most potent in whole, uncooked fruits, vegetables, and sprouts. (See chapter 3 for more details about antioxidants and living foods.)

LONG-TERM STUDIES

As in many scientific endeavors, we can currently turn only to animal studies to draw long-term conclusions about a health practice. The most remarkable of these studies in the field of living foods is one published by Francis Pottenger, Jr., M.D., in his *Pottenger's Cats*.[13] This report detailed the results of a ten-year diet study of six hundred cats. The results showed the destructive effects of cooked foods (diet-deficient foods) and the health-promoting effects of raw foods (optimum-diet foods) across generations. The results speak for themselves:

First Generation Diet-Deficient Cats
Heart problems; nearsightedness, farsightedness; under activity of the thyroid or inflammation of the thyroid gland; infection of the kidney, of the liver, of the testes, of the ovaries; arthritis, inflammation of the joints; inflammation of the nervous system with paralysis and meningitis.

Second Generation Diet-Deficient Cats
These cats are the kittens born to females of the first deficient generation. All symptoms have become progressively worse from one generation to the next. Much more irritable, dangerous to handle, sex interest is slack or perverted, role reversal, allergies, and skin lesions.

Abortion in pregnant females is common, running about 25 percent in the first deficient generation to about 70 percent in the second generation. Deliveries are generally difficult with many females dying in labor. The mortality rate of the kittens also is high as the kittens are either born dead or born too frail to nurse.

Third Generation Diet-Deficient Cats
These cats are the kittens born to females of the second generation eating a deficient diet.

There are never more than three generations of deficient cats because of the third generations' inability to produce healthy viable offspring.

By the time the third deficient generation is born, the cats are so bankrupt that none survive beyond the sixth month of life, thereby terminating the strain.

Optimum-Diet Cats

The cats fed a diet of ⅔ raw meat, ⅓ raw milk and cod liver oil show striking uniformity in their sizes and their skeletal developments. From generation to generation they maintain a regular, broad face with prominent maler and orbital arches, adequate nasal cavities, broad dental arches and regular dentition. The configuration of the female skull is different from the male skull and each sex maintains its distinct anatomical features. The membranes are firm and of good, pink color with no evidence of infection or degenerative change.

To finish the experiment, Dr. Pottenger studied plants fertilized by manure from the two groups of cats. The plants with the raw-food manure grew excellently. The plants fed the cooked-food manure were weak and struggled to survive, highlighting the lack of any life-giving features in the cooked-food diet.

THESE ARE THE FACTS

From animals to humans, the idea that the body can easily digest and assimilate cooked food properly may someday prove to be the most harmful assumption of science. There's no doubt that cooking reduces vitamin and mineral availability; destroys enzymes, hormones, and oxygen; promotes acid accumulation in the body; interferes with thorough digestion; and weakens the immune system and the bioactive electrical charge of the body's tissues and cells. It also weakens the power of naturally occurring antioxidants. In sum, cooking is greatly responsible for the toxic dump sites we've created within our bodies.

Living foods clean up these dump sites; they cleanse clogged systems, restore good health and vitality to all body cells, and give us personal control over our health and longevity. These are the facts of living foods.

3

Living Longer and Better: A Program for Physical Health

Of all the many thousands of species on Earth, only humans cook and process foods, and only humans are so penalized with poor health and rapid aging. Diet alone has caused an epidemic of disease, pain, and suffering that is entirely preventable; this truly is a human tragedy.

We can't wholly blame our present state of poor health on lack of vitamins, minerals, protein, fiber, or calories because modern foods are routinely "fortified" with these nutrients and most people eat too much food, not too little. We are, however, malnourished in enzymes, hormones, oxygen, alkaline foods, and bioactive materials. These things are required to build and fortify blood, bones, nerves, organs, and tissues and to maintain healthy digestive and immune systems. The influence on health of these components of living food is so dramatic that reams of research and my own experience make it possible for me to state emphatically that there is no physical ailment known today that can not be arrested or improved with the Hippocrates Health Program.

Living foods have been used with great success to heal arthritis, high blood pressure, menstrual difficulties, obesity, cancer, chronic fatigue syndrome, allergies, diabetes, ulcers, heart and other circulatory diseases, hormone disturbances, diverticulosis, anemia, a weak immune system, and many other ailments and degenerative diseases.

Like all vegetarian diets, a living-foods diet improves health and well-being by eliminating meat and dairy products. This first step automatically cleans the veins and arteries of fat and reduces the buildup of protein deposits. But unlike other vegetarians, living-food vegetarians thrive on the health-promoting components of oxygen, bioelectricity, enzymes, hormones, and alkalinity found in uncooked and unprocessed foods.

Chapter 2 explained why these factors have encouraged living-food vegetarians to take a giant step beyond macrobiotics and vegan-vegetarianism, but knowing how something works in theory isn't as convincing as seeing it work in real life. This chapter will tell you stories of living-food vegetarians who have found healing, recovery, and optimal health through the Hippocrates Health Program and are delighted to share their experiences with you.

HERE'S TO A LONG AND HEALTHY LIFE

How sad that we have been conditioned to think of ailments such as osteoporosis, cardiovascular disease, arthritis, and senility as part of growing old—in other words, as expected and normal! This acceptance of disease-riddled aging turns a myth with no scientific backbone into a self-fulfilling prophesy. Yes, we will all eventually die. But there's no reason we cannot remain active, sharp, alert, productive, and healthy until that time. Aging is not synonymous with disease and infirmity.

It's not added years that cause the body to age into a diseased state. It's the cell starvation that results from years of ingesting processed and cooked foods. Such foods are stripped of their life, and they do not supply what the body needs to function efficiently for a long period of time. In fact, they wear down the body by turning the body chemistry highly acidic. This places an enormous strain on the liver and kidneys as they try to process the calcium, magnesium, potassium, and sodium that the acid pulls from the muscles and nerve cells. It seems the human body is able to cope with this diet during youth because of its incredible resiliency. But eventually such a diet takes a heavy toll, and mature age becomes fraught with severe physical problems.

But that does not mean that the body falls apart by internal design. In fact, many medical and nutritional scientists believe that with proper maintenance, no healthy 20-year-old should die before age 70. Those who live past 70 should expect to remain physically and mentally active until around their 140th birthday. Why not? We have no more reason to accept the average American male life expectancy of 72 than do Russian males who have an average life expectancy of 57. Just because these figures state today's averages doesn't mean they're the upper limit.

This conclusion is backed not only by many gerontologists, but by current demographics. More and more Americans are hitting three-digit ages. A spokesperson for the Population Reference Bureau Inc., a private research group, recently told me that fifty-two thousand Americans are age 100 or older, and the number of American centenarians may reach one million by the middle of the twenty-first century. We have proof that the body does not need to wear out before its hundredth birthday, but the question now remains, how can we make these extended years fruitful, productive, and healthy? Someone who lives to the ripe old age of 105 but is hooked up to tubes, wires, and a respirator has not quite found the fountain of youth. The secret to healthy aging is not in pharmaceuticals, surgical procedures, or exotic, alchemical formulas; it is in the food we put on our plates.

When we accede to nature's plan for us to eat only vegetables, fruits, seeds, nuts, and grains, we increase our chances of reaping the benefits of old age that nature intended. At one time, before the recent massive move into unnatural diets, people aged gracefully, gaining wisdom and knowledge along the way. Those reaching the centennial mark were more alive in their incisive awareness and enlightenment than 20-year-olds.

The young did not fear the thought of aging, but respected and understood the significant contribution of their elders, holding them in high esteem. The elderly did not feel unwanted and disengaged because they had their physical and mental health, which allowed them to contribute to and enhance their society.

How can we go on as a culture if we live with the expectation that we will all eventually become infirm, chronically ill, and/or incapacitated statistics of the health-care system? We will go on because in the twenty-first century more and more of us will embrace the Hippocrates lifestyle and diet. The change will offer us fuel that feeds the body's cells with oxygen, enzymes, and bioelectrical strength, which keeps tissues and cells clear of acidic debris, and so keeps the immune and digestive systems strong and functioning right to the end. This pampering of the body's biological needs is the true fountain of youth.

This is bad news for the growing geriatric industry that is sitting in wait for the baby-boomers to age into infirmity. But it is great news for you!

Aging: A Comparative Tale of Eighty-Three-Year-Old Twins

When eighty-three-year-old identical twins, Harry and Thomas Bromley, were guests at Hippocrates, their presence stimulated quite a bit of interest and curiosity. Although they were difficult to tell apart in their twenties, their differing lifestyles had brought about a marked physiological change in later years that made quite a difference in their appearance.

For the past sixty years, Harry has been a health-conscious vegetarian. A picture of health, Harry practices yoga and walks between two and five miles a day; he does breathing exercises and swims. With an exuberant personality and social life, Harry enjoys each day; he dates and dances often (kidding that he has to find younger women in their sixties who can keep up with him). Harry enjoys being alive.

Thomas, on the other hand, is an avowed junk-food eater—he lives on burgers, pizzas, colas, meat, and potatoes. His appearance typifies the deterioration that is caused by a long-term, non-nutritious, anything-goes diet. He is overweight, sluggish, and suffering chronic health problems.

The most pronounced difference between these brothers is in their degree of mental sharpness. Harry is bright and energetic, an avid reader, and an animated conversationalist with the mental acuity of someone half his age. Thomas has trouble remembering things; he lacks self-confidence and is very dependent on his brother.

In all of Hippocrates' history, this was the first time we saw such a striking comparison. Harry stood proudly as an example of the benefits of long-time adherence to a good, nutritious diet. Thomas sat feebly, like a poster child for the average American diet of highly-processed foods, snacks with too much sugar or salt, and a wide variety of fast foods that are high in fat and cholesterol and low in dietary fiber and nutrition.

CANCER

The statistics are startling! According to the American Cancer Society:

- Cancer is the second most common cause of death in the U.S. today.
- 1 out of 3 Americans alive today will develop cancer.
- Within five years, 2 out of every 5 Americans will develop cancer.

What's going on? Well, we know that cancer is caused when normal, healthy cells mutate into abnormal, cancerous cells that propagate and spread. But what makes them mutate to begin with? For years, researchers have struggled against the clock to find the trigger. In some cases the key seems to lie in genetically inherited, predisposed genes that cause cancer when switched on by some external aggravant. In other cases, environmental toxins such as asbestos and smog are the culprits. We also know that free radicals, which are the result of a poor lifestyle, are one of the major contributing factors in the development of cancer. Also, xenoestrogens from synthetic chemicals turn into estrogen and contribute to the cancer crisis. And we've learned without doubt that cigarette smoke causes lung cancer.

Now that scientific study has proven the connection between cancer and external triggers, the link between cancer and food falls right into place; yet so many people refuse to accept that what they put in their mouths can result in cancerous tumors. Maybe this resistance has much to do with the suspect foods being mom's home cooking and barbecue favorites.

The Support of Scientific Literature

The evidence is indisputable—a representative of the American Cancer Society estimates that diet and nutrition can be named in 30 percent to 40 percent of cancer cases. A quick tour through any medical database will bring up reams of studies—one after the other attesting to the link between diet and cancer. Consider these few:

- "Diet and Colon Cancer" (Research report) by E. Giovannucci, *Cancer Researcher Weekly,* Dec. 13, 1993, p. 21.
- "Animal Fat Linked to Prostate Cancer" (Study of 47,855 men, which found that those who ate large amounts of red meat were 80 percent more likely to contract prostate cancer.) *Facts on File,* Oct. 14, 1993, p. 774.
- "Dietary Factors and the Risk of Endometrial Cancer" (Periodical report) *Cancer Researcher Weekly,* July 19, 1993, p. 26.
- "Diet Versus Cancer" (Diets high in vegetables, fruits, and grains reduce risk of cancer according to this study by the American Cancer Society) *New York Times,* October 7, 1992, p. B7.
- "Studies Create Confusion, But Eating Greens Is Good" (National Cancer Institute and Johns Hopkins University School of Medicine

studies on health benefits of eating vegetables) by Wayne Hearn, *American Medical News,* May 9, 1994, p. 20.

Phytochemicals in Living Foods Ward Off Cancer

The new buzzword when discussing nutrition and cancer is *phyto-chemicals.* Phytochemicals are components within natural food that have been proven to retard cancer development and growth. One such substance is sulforaphane, which researchers from Johns Hopkins University School of Medicine extracted from broccoli and gave to rats that already had been treated with a carcinogen that causes mammary tumors. The substance (also found in cauliflower, brussels sprouts, turnips, and kale) significantly reduced the size and number of the tumors and delayed their development. The researchers say the substances enhance the performance of enzymes that protect against cancer-causing agents.[1]

Actually, phytochemicals work at several steps in the process of cancer development. "At almost every one of the steps along the pathway leading to cancer," says epidemiologist John Potter of the University of Minnesota, "there are one or more compounds in vegetables or fruit that will slow up or reverse the process."[2] Take a look at this sampling:

Broccoli   also contains *phenethyl isothiocyanate,* which prevents carcinogens from binding to DNA, and *indole-3-carbinol,* which causes estrogen to break down into a harmless metabolite rather than the form linked to breast cancer.

Cabbage   harbors a high concentration of *indole-3-carbinol* along with *oltipraz,* which increases enzymes that protect against a wide range of cancers and *brassinin,* which has been shown to protect against mammary and skin tumors.

Garlic and onions   contain *allylic sulfides,* which work by waking up enzymes that detoxify cancer-causing chemicals inside cells.

Chili peppers   contain *capsaicin,* which keeps toxic molecules (especially those in cigarette smoke) from attaching to DNA—the spot where sparks ignite into lung and other cancers.

Citrus fruits and berries   are storehouses of *flavonoids,* which keep cancer-causing hormones from latching onto a cell.

Soybeans   contain *genistein,* which seems to keep tiny tumors from connecting to capillaries that carry oxygen and nutrition. This may explain why Japanese men who relocate to the West and adapt to a low-soy diet have a significantly increased rate of prostate cancer.

Tomatoes   are rich in *p-coumaric acid* and *chlorogenic acid* that block the formation of nitrosamine compounds, which are strongly linked to stomach, liver, and bladder cancer. Strawberries, pineapples, and peppers are also rich in these acids.

The research into phytochemicals recently took a major step forward during a conference in Washington, D.C., with doctors, college professors, and researchers from around the world attending and lecturing. The National Cancer Institute has launched a multimillion-dollar project to find, isolate, and study phytochemicals. The National Cancer Institute, the American Cancer Society, and many other medical authorities now agree that living, fresh fruits and vegetables are important in warding off cancer.

Cancer-Causing Foods?

Research has found that the most notable carcinogens are found in cooked, fried foods and high-protein foods.

Cooked foods.   Cooking foods disrupts their RNA and DNA structure, destroys most of the nutritive value of fats, creates carcinogenic and mutagenic structures in fats, and produces free radicals.

A free radical is a molecule that's missing an electron. As you may recall from high school chemistry class, molecules like to stay in balance; one that's missing an electron desperately wants to rebalance its electrical charge by stealing an electron from wherever it can. When free radicals are loose in the body, they can steal electrons from molecules of fat, protein, or even DNA in cells. Altered DNA can lead a cell to mutate and reproduce uncontrollably. We call this cancer.

The body defends itself against free radicals with an array of enzymes that repair damaged cells and break down the free radicals into water and harmless oxygen. This natural defense process is sabotaged when we eat cooked foods because cooking increases the number of free radicals and reduces the number of enzymes supplied to the body.

To fight cancer, the body needs those enzymes that are wiped out during the cooking process. In fact, the world-renowned professor and doctor from Vienna, Dr. Warba, states that enzymes are a new approach to cancer treatment. Two main factors influence the treatment of cancer cells: defense of the host, and virulence of the cancer cells. Enzymes in living foods address both these factors. They improve the defense mechanism in the body by lowering the virulence of the cancerous cells. Dr. Warba feels that this causes modulation of the cell membrane, uncovers the cell surface and receptors, improves immunity, and reduces the stickiness of the tumor cells.[3]

We also know that there are genes in the body whose enzymes guard against cancer by preventing the various cell changes that lead to malignancy. Researchers at the Department of Microbiology and Immunology at the Jefferson Cancer Institute, for example, have recently identified a gene whose enzyme prevents the growth of intestinal polyps, a precursor to colon cancer. Researcher Linda Siracusa says that the enzyme may play an important role during fat metabolism, working to block the harmful effects of fat on the lining of the intestines. Another possibility is that the enzyme may help eliminate certain types of bacteria associated with a high-fat diet. Or, the enzyme may work to directly eliminate abnormal cells.[4] Whatever the exact mechanism, it is certain that efficiently functioning enzymes can stop cancer in its tracks.

To further illustrate the dangers of cooked foods, the American Cancer Society reports: "Recent studies have demonstrated that high-temperature cooking of meat gives rise to a wide variety of substances that have been shown to cause cancer in animals and that have caused damage to DNA in well-established test systems. The toxic action is considered to be a prelude to cancer."[5] To support this, a 1990 study at the National Cancer Institute led by Richard Adamson, Ph.D., found very potent mutagens known as heterocyclic aromatic amines (HAAs) in highly heated beef, fish, and poultry. These HAAs are among the most powerful mutagens ever studied, meaning that even a relatively small amount can cause significant damage to DNA.[6] (Mutagens are almost always carcinogenic.)

New research from the Lawrence Livermore National Laboratories in Livermore, California, indicates that it's not just highly heated meats that pose a problem. Lab scientist Mark Knize and a team of researchers studied the effects of different cooking methods on a variety of foods, including breads, rice, eggs, tofu, and gluten- and tofu-based vegetable patties. Using a test that is designed to mimic human metabolism, the researchers found mutagens in each of the cooked foods. In almost every instance, the higher the heat, the higher the level of mutagens.[7]

Protein. The Center for Science in the Public Interest reports that the average American takes in about 150 grams of protein each day. But you need only a fraction of that amount. Where does the excess go? Well, the body can't store protein. So when a diet supplies blood and cells with too much protein, the lymphatic system attempts to remove the excess. But when the burden becomes too great for the lymph to handle, protein "traps" (tumors) are created, which the body seals off in order to protect the rest of its organs and tissues. As Nobel prize winner Dr. Otto Warburg showed, when oxygen supply is decreased by as little as 30 percent, these trapped cells can become malignant cancer cells. Warburg found that, unlike normal healthy cells, malignant cancer cells don't require oxygen to reproduce. In a sense, the cancerous cells consume waste, saving the body from poisoning by excess protein. But this survival tactic can cause uncontrolled, terminal cancer.[8]

Unfortunately, our processed, cooked foods are dead; they contain no oxygen to keep the cells oxygen-rich. Obviously this leaves them open to mutation and malignancy. Living foods not only contain less protein, but they are an alkaline food that helps neutralize the highly acidic and toxic nitrogen released when the body tries to process excess protein.

Wheatgrass, a staple of the Hippocrates Health Program, is an example of a living food with proven cancer-fighting properties, according to Dr. Pnina Bar-Sella. Her 1995 study reported on the antimutagenic activities of the chlorophyll found in wheat-sprout extracts. The results: "Chlorophyll has been determined to be the major active factor in wheat sprout extract that inhibits the mutagenic effect of carcinogens requiring metabolic activation. The findings were confirmed by the testing of equivalent commercial compounds."[9]

Another study of the relationship between diet and cancer in mice by Arthur B. Robinson and colleagues at the Oregon Institute of Science and Medicine in 1994 found protein reduction to be a major factor in cancer suppression. Dr. Robinson reported, "Apparently, low protein in the raw fruit and vegetable diet is a significant factor in reduction of cancer growth rate."[10]

Many physicians who study this relationship are changing their own eating habits. Dr. Charles Simone, director of the Protective Cancer Center in Lawrenceville, New Jersey, began studying the links between diet and cancer in 1983 and hasn't had a hamburger or slice of pizza since. He's also convinced his family. "You could not entice my children with any hamburger or ice cream or cake," he boasts.[11] The evidence is that strong.

Breast Cancer

It's quite clear that a diet rich in animal products and oxygen-deficient cooked foods significantly raises the risk of cancer. This has been made especially clear in the studies linking diet to breast cancer, which strikes hundreds of thousands of women worldwide (roughly 182,000 women in the U.S. alone each year!). In fact, a direct correlation can be drawn between a country's animal fat consumption and the number of breast cancer cases (probably because fat tissue can make estrogen). How amazing to find that the development of breast cancer is avoidable—a choice based on what we choose to put in our mouths. (Men are not spared the ravages of the diet-cancer connection either. Animal products are turned into male hormones called androgens, which stimulate the prostate gland. After decades of running androgens through this gland, it's not surprising that it becomes enlarged and cancerous.)

In addition to the relationship between cancer and animal fat, new studies are zeroing in on the link between synthetic, hormone-mimicking compounds (called xenoestrogens, or foreign estrogens) found in certain pesticides, drugs, fuels, and plastics. Researchers Devra Davis and H. Leon Bradlow from the Strang-Cornell Cancer Research Laboratory in New York propose that increased exposure to xenoestrogens may explain the rise in the incidence of breast cancer over the past several decades in many nations. They also believe that the compounds contribute to a range of reproductive disorders that have reportedly become increasingly common in men worldwide—notably testicular cancer, undescended testes, urinary tract defects, and lowered sperm counts.[12]

The cells in our bodies do react to external stimulation, both bad and good. When we eat foods laden with fat and chemical preservatives, additives, and pesticides, we contribute to their transformation into deadly tumors.

The following true story is a remarkable tale of bravery in the face of "terminal" breast cancer. It is an amazing story that is just one of the hundreds like it I could tell you.

Breast Cancer: A Journey to Health

By Rachel Budnick

My health crisis started in May of 1988. I wasn't feeling well and one morning I woke up to discover that something itched in my breast. I scratched it and felt a little ball. I called my doctor and made an appointment for the same day. I had previously had a lot of benign cysts and my New York doctor would remove the fluid by injection. But I had recently moved to Chicago and had an interim doctor who said I had to go for a mammogram.

The technicians took a lot of pictures, and the nurse looked grim. When I asked what was wrong, the radiologist said he couldn't tell me, but that I should have had a mammogram years ago. This was the very beginning of my saga.

When I decided to go back to my doctor in New York, my Chicago physician gave me a sealed note with the word "Personal" written on the outside. I opened the note and found out that he thought the lump was malignant.

The New York doctor said I had to go for another mammogram, so I did, thinking maybe the first one had been wrong. He removed the fluid from the lump and sent it to the lab to be tested. The results came back positive. Then my doctor said I should go for a biopsy.

I went back to Chicago and found a doctor I trusted at the University of Chicago who did the biopsy. A few days later, he gave me the final word: the lump was malignant; I had something called infiltrated ductile carcinoma.

He said I should have a mastectomy. First, I went to other specialists for second and third opinions, but they all told me the same thing. One specialist at Northwestern University even suggested that since the cancer had infiltrated the entire breast, I would be wise to have both breasts removed at the same time and save myself a second trip to the hospital! Reconstructive plastic surgery was also recommended.

I had found the lump in the beginning of May. Within two weeks, I had had the biopsy, and a week later I was scheduled to go in for surgery. I was told that when the growth is exposed to air it grows much faster (which is why they like to operate soon after the biopsy). It was true. From a pea-sized growth, my lump grew to the size of my fist.

That's when I started looking for an alternative. I called all over the world. I tried to contact people who had some experience in alternative ways of dealing with cancer because I was looking for someone who wouldn't insist on surgery. But I could not find anyone to talk to who had survived breast cancer without surgery. So I decided I was going to be a pioneer.

Finally, a few days before my scheduled surgery, I found the Hippocrates Institute in West Palm Beach, Florida. I called and said I wanted to come down right away. I'd made up my mind.

Meanwhile, friends and do-gooders called to wish me luck with my surgery and were shocked to hear about my decision. "What are you doing?" they yelled. They were absolutely certain I was committing suicide. But I just wanted to get out of Chicago and start on the program. That's when I started to get well.

I stayed at Hippocrates for five weeks because I wanted to learn the whole program. But I soon discovered that even five weeks is just a drop in the bucket. I was really sick. I was extremely stressed out, and I had a lot of detoxing to do. It was tough, but within the first fourteen days, the tumor began to shrink. When I left the institute, I was on my way, but it took a long time. Recovery is a gradual process. Five months later, I returned to Hippocrates for another visit. In the sixth month, the tumor was completely gone.

I started feeling better very gradually. I would have a few good hours out of a week. Then I graduated to feeling normal one day a week, and eventually the number of good days outnumbered the bad.

I also benefited from the Hippocrates Program in other ways besides ridding myself of cancer. My energy level is now much higher, my skin has improved tremendously, my hair has almost doubled in volume, my nails are stronger, and my skin tone is much, much better. I still continue the program religiously and remain cancer-free eight years after my first visit.

HEART DISEASE

The heart is subject to two forms of debility: hardening of the arteries and enlargement. The first condition is not really a hardening of the arteries at all; it's more a narrowing called atherosclerosis. This results from a buildup of cholesterol or plaque on the insides of the arteries and veins, forcing the heart to labor excessively to get the blood through unnaturally small channels. The condition is usually accompanied by high blood pressure. If the plaque builds up on the walls of the arteries feeding blood to the heart and blocks the blood flow, that part of the heart dependent on the blocked-off artery will die. This is called a myocardial infarction, or heart attack. Animal fats and animal products are the main contributors to arterial plaque buildup.

Heart attacks are by far the largest cause of death globally today. According to a representative at the American Heart Association, every twenty seconds another person is stricken. Every minute another person dies. What a tragedy to learn that there would be no such thing as heart attacks if the blood were allowed to flow freely and easily through the coronary arteries.

The enlarged heart is another preventable cardiac condition. Remember, the heart is a muscle. Like all muscles, it needs a constant supply of fresh oxygen and nutrients. The flow of blood that feeds the heart must be supercharged with nutrients; without proper nourishment, the heart muscle weakens causing it to lose its elasticity and strength and become flabby and enlarged. It's not surprising that a diet comprised of excessive amounts of soft drinks, alcohol, coffee, drugs, stimulants, refined flour products, and highly processed foods results in an enlarged heart.

As early as 1961, the *Journal of the American Medical Association* stated that 90 percent to 97 percent of heart disease could be prevented by a vegetarian diet.[13] The reason for this is not a mystery. Animal products contain high levels of cholesterol, which is the clogging agent responsible for blocking blood flow. No grain, vegetable, nut, seed, fruit, legume, or vegetable oil contains cholesterol—not one. Obviously, anyone who knows this and yet continues on an animal fat diet is choosing an early death. Imagine having such a choice: "Behind Door Number 1 is a steak and an early death. Behind Door Number 2 is a feast of vegetables and fruits and a long healthy life. Which do you choose?" Apparently the choice is not so easy—the number one cause of death is still heart disease.

The medical community contributes to this wayward choice by setting recommended cholesterol levels that are much too high. "Average" levels are anything between 160 and 330. As Dr. John McDougall, author of *The McDougall Plan,* has noted: "The average male in our society has a greater than 50 percent chance of dying from a heart attack. Under these circumstances, no consolation should be gained from being average."[14] Nathan Pritikin, author of *The Pritikin Program for Diet and Exercise,* recognized this same problem saying, "Every so-called 'normal' level in our country is guaranteed to close arteries. 'Normal' in our country simply means that you can walk from one room to another."[15]

A healthy cholesterol level should be 100 plus your age to a maximum of 150. Achieving this level on a diet of living foods is not a struggle; it happens automatically.

Heart Attacks: All in the Family

Gerard and Larry Aliseo spent many years working hard in their New Jersey family businesses: construction and food importing from Italy. Work was the most important thing for them—that is until at age thirty, older brother Larry had his first heart attack, followed by a second and a third at age thirty-one. Gerard's heart attack came two years later when he turned thirty-one.

Larry had a massive myocardial infarction, losing 50 percent of his heart muscle—the whole back of his heart had died. "I knew that nutrition was important to my recovery," says Larry, "so I went to a nutritionist and then I'd spend one year on a healthy diet and then two years off." All the while, he smoked, worked too much, and lugged around twenty-five extra pounds. His total cholesterol count was 360.

After the third heart attack, Larry put his health in the hands of medication; he was taking four different drugs, and he wore a nitroglycerin patch. The medications were making him feel awful. He was having nightmares, headaches, and was constantly tired. His prognosis was dire. Larry went back to his nutritionist who told him he had no more time to fool around; it was time to visit Hippocrates Institute.

At Hippocrates, Larry learned why his diet had set him up for his heart attacks and why he was leaving himself at risk for another. While at Hippocrates, his cholesterol went down to 200. He started to feel better.

Meanwhile Gerard was back in New Jersey still working and eating the wrong foods. "When Larry told me what he was doing, I thought he was a little kooky. After all, I had given up red meat and I thought that made me a healthy eater." Then he had his heart attack. He was luckier than his brother; Gerard lost only 8 percent of his heart muscle, but his "recovery" required eight pills a day that caused miserable side effects. It was getting harder to ignore his brother's good health. Larry had lost weight, felt good, and looked younger. Finally, Gerard went to Hippocrates. His cholesterol was 360 when he checked in; by the time he left, it had dropped to 181, and he was feeling much better.

Gerard (now age thirty-eight) and Larry (age forty-one) still come to Hippocrates several times a year. The Aliseo brothers are genetically predisposed to heart attacks—their father had his first one at fifty-three. Gerard points out that they had their heart attacks twenty years earlier than expected, but this reflects the deteriorating health of this generation.

Although they are still in the family business, Larry says he doesn't go to work in the morning until he has eaten a living-foods breakfast and relaxed his mind. He and his brother ride bicycles together eight miles a day. Larry is completely off medication; his doctor had no reason to keep him on pills as his radiant health precluded any need for pharmaceutical interference.

People see Larry and Gerard now and ask what happened—they look and feel great! It's no mystery what's caused the turnaround. "I was reckless before," admits Larry. "I put everything else before my own health. Now I want to be around my kids and teach them how to eat and live the Hippocrates way. When I think of how much earlier we had our heart attacks than our dad did, I wonder if my son will have a heart attack in his twenties. Kids need to know about the connection between what they eat and how long and how well they live. They can turn things around."

That's the amazing thing about atherosclerosis—it's preventable and reversible. The plaque that builds up over years of eating dead and fatty food will dissolve and completely disappear on a living-foods diet.

ARTHRITIS

Arthritis affects the lives of an estimated eleven million Americans. Often untreatable through conventional medical means, the chronic pain of arthritis reduces the sufferer's ability to perform daily tasks and it influences relationships with family, friends, colleagues, and even self. The annual cost of treatment and care and the losses in time, money, and productivity are colossal. But there is hope. By attending to the cause of arthritis through nutrition, you can live pain-free.

The word arthritis only broadly described the ailment. Like cancer, arthritis exists in many forms. The two most common, and the subject of this discussion are inflammatory arthritis and degenerative arthritis. Inflammatory arthritis generally designates a subgroup of arthritis characterized by inflammation of the joints. The most well known and most debilitating of these is rheumatoid arthritis. The process by which rheumatoid arthritis attacks the body is quite methodical and consistent. It first assaults the membrane that lines the joint (synovial membrane), causing inflammation. The inflamed membrane swells and covers the joint and progresses into the underlying cartilage; this interferes with the ability of the cartilage to form the gliding surfaces of the joint. Simultaneously, changes occur in the bone below the cartilage; the bone loses its mineral components and becomes fibrous; the deformed material also spreads to the cartilage. As the disease infiltrates the body's system, a bloodless fibrous tissue is formed that results in stiffness in the joint. Although brief periods of remission occur, the disease is progressive. The last and most crippling blow happens when the fibrous tissue becomes bone; this signals the end of the degenerative process. Pain and motion plateau at this time, neither increasing nor decreasing.

Degenerative arthritis (also called osteoarthritis) begins at the cartilage. The gliding surface of the cartilage flakes off. The process then destroys the binding material that holds together the bundles of cartilage fibers. We can think of the cartilage fibers as stacks of balanced pipes that had once been tied together; in weight-bearing joints these fibers soon are worn away, leaving only empty pits. Ultimately, all of the cartilage is worn away; the joint space disappears, and the bone surfaces are in direct contact with each other. Since the cartilage is a shock absorber for the joints, arthritic pain becomes more apparent as the cartilage is lost.

The Arthritis Foundation insists there is no relation between diet and arthritis. I predict they will change their position in the very near future—the facts are too strong to ignore.

The first highly publicized study came out of Wayne State University Medical School in Michigan. Here, six rheumatoid arthritis patients went on a fat-free diet. In seven weeks, all of the subjects showed total disappearance of their symptoms. When fats were reintroduced into their diets, it took only three days for the symptoms to reappear.[16]

Immediately on the heels of that study, another was reported in the British Medical Journal. This study focused on a thirty-eight-year-old woman who had been suffering from worsening rheumatoid arthritis for eleven years. Three weeks after she removed all dairy products from her diet, she showed signs of improvement. In four months, her arthritic symptoms had completely disappeared.[17]

How does diet affect arthritis? As new bone cells generate, their health is based on the amount of nutrition the body provides. A strong skeletal structure needs a full store of enzymes, amino acids, trace minerals, and trace elements as well as vitamins and healthy hormones. Malnourishment can be the core of arthritis.

As new bone cells are formed, they need plenty of oxygen-rich blood to grow healthy and strong. But if the body is full of fats, there isn't enough oxygen in the blood to build bones and joints. To aggravate the situation, the fat encapsulates the cells, making absorption of nutrients impossible.

Also, if the body is lacking minerals, the generation of new bone cells is weakened. High-protein diets rob the body of the minerals needed to maintain healthy bone structure; the protein actually will pull calcium out of the bones.

A diet low in essential nutrients, oxygen, and enzymes also turns the blood level acidic. Wastes from the high acid content become free radicals that aggravate the bone structure causing inflammation. This condition sets the stage for bone deposits and disintegration of bone joints.

A living-foods diet can prevent and/or relieve arthritis. It does this in a number of ways:

1. By reducing protein intake, it protects the body's cells from the loss of mineralization and the attack of free radicals.
2. It reduces systemic acidity. Processed and cooked foods raise the level of acid in the body, leaving it open to arthritis.
3. It gives the bone's cells easily absorbable nutrients, enzymes, and oxygen that they need to stay strong and healthy.
4. It adds extra enzymes that add an electrical charge to the bone's cells. This creates a physical attraction between the cells that can actually break up the arthritic blockages and deposits and strengthen the renewing bone. In redeveloping new bone structure, the enzymes unify the bone structure and bond the pits and holes.

Rheumatoid Arthritis: "Like a Gigantic Toothache"

Ellie Oster is a vibrant, active woman who was once completely crippled with rheumatoid arthritis. When she arrived at Hippocrates Health Institute, she had been fighting the disease for ten painful years. Her difficult experience began when she awoke one morning with an excruciating ache in her back. She went to a chiropractor but found that he was unable to help her. Soon her right leg became paralyzed, and it was then that Ellie began to realize that she had a very serious disease indeed, one that was creeping into every part of her body.

Ellie was diagnosed with rheumatoid arthritis and was in unimaginable pain all the time. "It was like having a gigantic toothache all over," she remembers. "Such pain drives you right up the wall." After a year of watching her knees swell up like grapefruits and being confined to bed most of the time with a daily intake of twenty-five aspirins, she went to New York City where, at Columbia Presbyterian Hospital, she began the long road of treatment prescribed for rheumatoid arthritics: plenty of hot packs, warm water, and exercise. Since Ellie did not feel that pain killers would help heal the source of her arthritis, she refused them, opting instead to swim up to three or four hours a day in her own heated, 90-degree pool. She saw this treatment as a prison sentence she had to serve. And so she did.

But at the end of ten years, she had not improved. Her doctor felt that she was at the end of her rope; Ellie was totally enfeebled, literally frozen. The doctor himself was losing patience with her and wanted to pump her full of drugs. But her instincts would not let Ellie give in to drugs. At the time when she needed it most, she heard about Hippocrates.

It seems that Ellie's daughter-in-law had a friend who said she had been healed of cancer through the Hippocrates Program and came to talk with Ellie. As Ellie listened, the same inner voice that had been refusing drugs said, "This is it." And so she came to the institute, determined to stay an entire month. What a shock it must have been!

Before she arrived at the Institute, her health habits had been dreadful; like many people, she smoked, drank cocktails, consumed coffee, sugar, salt, meat and dairy products, indeed all of the things the institute's health rebuilding program excludes. It was quite frightening to be left with only a plateful of greens. But Ellie wanted to get well. She was tired of being half a person physically, emotionally, and spiritually. Luckily, the program made sense to her. Assimilation of nutrients and elimination of wastes are the keys to good health. What could be more logical?

At the end of her first two weeks, Ellie slept soundly for the first time in years. But as she went through detoxification, she was also very sick and very frightened. She remembers sobbing and crying over the phone to her husband, wanting desperately to go back home, but feeling so weak that she couldn't even get her clothes on, or her things packed, or her luggage out to a cab. Yet, once she passed through this healing crisis, she felt a resurgence of vitality. She knew that she was going to live—and this time as a whole person. Fifty percent of the pain she'd been enduring for ten years disappeared after one month.

Ellie remained on the program 100 percent for two more years. She feels this strict adherence is very important and absolutely necessary for the body to fully heal itself. Such devout concentration paid off. She got well. Her doctor was incredulous, but he could not deny what he saw for himself, and since then he, too, has turned to living foods.

Ellie has not had arthritic pain in twenty years. She swims a half hour every morning and evening. Although she no longer has to stay on the living-foods program, she does so anyway. She feels it uplifts her physically, emotionally, and spiritually.

Ellie, who is now well into her eighties, enjoys sharing her wonderful transformation with others. Recently she spoke at a convention of senior citizens in Atlantic City, New Jersey. The advice she gives others is this: "Go on a living-foods diet, exercise regularly, and have faith in the power of the body to heal itself."

IMMUNE POWER

The immune system is on call twenty-four hours a day; it is ready to attack any foreign invader that threatens good health. In theory, it should be at rest most of the time and launching forceful attacks only when the system is threatened by disease-carrying bacteria, viruses, or fungi. But in the majority of today's population, the immune system works around the clock, kicking white blood cells into the bloodstream to defend us against what it thinks are unwelcomed substances—additives, pesticides, chemically-based supplements, and cooked foods. The result is a stressed and worn-out immune system that is barely able to do its real job when disease or infection appears. The chronically weakened immune system is the culprit in many of today's "incurable" medical dilemmas: chronic fatigue syndrome, HIV, multiple sclerosis, diabetes, cancer, heart disease, and so on.

The following "hopeless" cases will give you an idea of how diet can restore the body's ability to find balance and strength.

Infection: A Determined Fashion Model

Heather Miller was a twenty-five-year-old model in England making $200,000 a year. She lost a leg in a bizarre accident when a police motorcycle went out of control and ran her down as she stood on the sidewalk. Her recovery was slow and difficult; almost every day after the amputation, the stump had to be pierced or opened to release the pus. A few weeks after the accident, Heather had another operation to take three more inches off the stump in an attempt to stop the spread of the infection. But soon the infection returned. "The infection in my stump was really getting me down," remembers Heather. "Nothing seemed to be working, and antibiotics were no help. It got to the stage where I was terrified doctors would have to carry on operating just to keep the infection at bay."

That's when Heather headed to the Hippocrates Institute. "I'd heard of Hippocrates from a friend who had breast cancer," says

Heather. "She went there as a last resort, but after three months she was well. It's hard to believe, but it's true. So I thought I'd give it a try. After all, I had nothing to lose, apart from more of my stump. After just one week there, I knew it was the best move I'd ever made. Four days there did what four months of antibiotics and a new operation failed to do. It sounds a little crazy, but it works, and if it works, you can't knock it. It's like the elixir of life for me. I feel fantastic."

Candida Albicans

Candida albicans is a yeast product that grows inside all of us. Normally, its growth is controlled by bacteria in the intestines. But because pharmaceutical and animal-product antibiotics are so rampant in our society, the bacteria needed to patrol *Candida albicans* is often wiped out, allowing the yeast to invade and colonize in the body tissue. *Candida* causes varying symptoms including lethargy, chronic diarrhea, constipation, yeast vaginitis, bladder infections, menstrual cramps, asthma, migraine headaches, and severe depression.

   Candida is an opportunistic bacteria that will often invade a weakened person. Many patients with cancer, diabetes, cardiovascular illnesses, and other ailments also suffer the presence of *Candida,* making it much more difficult to become healthy again. Because of its varied effects, *Candida* is often misdiagnosed, leaving patients fruitlessly treating symptoms without ever touching on the root cause.

   Candida albicans is becoming more well known and more frequently diagnosed, but the prescribed treatments are still in question. Some of the worst advice regarding treatment through diet is the recommendation that the patient avoid anything with life in it and increase intake of animal foods. Through my practice, research, and findings with this disease, the opposite recommendation is what is needed. If you can imagine the internal body when infected with *Candida* as a dank, moldy, dripping cave, you would have a rather accurate picture. When one has an enzyme-deficient diet starving tissues of oxygen, the environment is perfect for this yeast to multiply.

The most effective way to clean up and rejuvenate the affected internal areas is to expose the body to sunlight and to eat a diet of raw, unprocessed vegetables, germinated seeds, grains, and nuts. Living foods maintain a healthy balance of bacteria and *Candida albicans*. The diet also cleanses body tissues where *Candida* has colonized. The proper balance of yeast and bacteria in the intestine and body "miraculously" heals physical and emotional problems that plague many people for years and years.

Some 25 percent of the people who attend the Hippocrates Institute are infected with this problem. We have found that the living-foods diet is a truly effective treatment, but even in the best-case scenario, it takes approximately a year and a half to regulate the system. If you suspect your ill health may be caused by *Candida albicans*, investigate further by having your blood tested at an immunological blood-testing facility that has a competent test procedure for *Candida*.

No Job, No Energy, No Explanation

"Six years ago," says Marilyn Canes, "so many doctors had told me that there was nothing wrong with me that I was ready to agree that my problem was all in my head. What else could it be?" Marilyn was so fatigued, that she quit her job after finding it impossible to get through the day without putting her head down on her desk and falling sound asleep. "People in my office thought I was drinking," she remembers. "I could barely walk from one end of the room to the other without losing my balance and needing a rest." So there she was—no job, no energy, no explanation.

That's when Marilyn heard about the Hippocrates Health Institute and came for a visit. By the end of her three week visit, Marilyn's energy had returned, her chronic vaginal infection was gone, her self-esteem was back, and her ailment had a name: *Candida albicans*.

Today, Marilyn is still a living-foods vegetarian and is still free of *Candida*. She returns to the institute every year—it's not only a peaceful retreat for her, but it reminds her of why living foods are her salvation from a life of pain, fatigue, and self-loathing.

ANTIOXIDANTS

The antioxidants found in living foods are surely partly responsible for the good health of all the followers of the Hippocrates Health Program. These substances found naturally in living fruits and vegetables battle the infamous free radicals that roam the body damaging cells and causing a long list of diseases and ailments.

Actually, researchers have determined that free radicals benefit the body by working with the immune system to ward off disease by killing alien bacteria and other invaders that enter your body. Also, they help regulate the contraction of the smooth muscles of your blood vessels and contribute to the control of your blood flow by improving the tone of the tissue lining of your vessels.[18]

Free radicals are released during the normal metabolism of your body, as your food is turned into energy by your body's cells. Your body's defense systems exist to keep the output of free radicals in balance. The problem arises when too many free radicals are generated for your internal antioxidant police force. When that happens, the radicals become renegades linked to many serious diseases and conditions including the following: premature aging, heart disease, immunodeficiency, arthritis, cancer, cataracts, allergies, and diabetes.

Normally, we have protective shields available in the form of antioxidants. A living-foods diet gives the body an abundant daily supply of these health warriors. The most celebrated of the antioxidants are the carotenoids. There are approximately forty of these substances, which are most potent in blocking cancer, fighting allergies, and slowing the aging process. They are found in carrots, sprouts, apricots, sweet potatoes, spinach, celery, squash, red peppers, tomatoes, oranges, and kale.

The most powerful members of the antioxidant family are the flavonoids, which are twenty times more potent than vitamin C and fifty times more active than vitamin E. Flavonoids protect against capillary damage, bruising, and improve overall immunity to heart disease and cancer. The best sources for flavonoids are onions, peppers, and selected herbs such as peppermint, spearmint, winter mint, and basil.

Vitamin C contains the antioxidant ascorbic acid. This can slow the onset of Parkinson's disease, reduce the risk of hardening of the arteries by increasing the amount of protective high-density lipo-protein (HDL) cholesterol in your bloodstream, help prevent cataracts by guarding the eyes against oxidation, help lower blood pressure, and protect against a wide spectrum of cancers. Vitamin C is found in parsley, sprouts, citrus fruits, kiwi, red peppers, cabbage, and leafy greens.

Vitamin E (tocopherol) is a fat-soluble vitamin-antioxidant and important immune system stimulant that helps alleviate fatigue and gives tissues oxygen to accelerate the healing of wounds, burns, and skin disorders such as acne and eczema. In partnership with the mineral selenium, it neutralizes free radicals that accelerate cellular and cerebral aging and raise the risk of cancer. Vitamin E is found in nuts and seeds, nut oils, wheat, and other grain sprouts.

Good herbal antioxidants to sip or sniff include alfalfa, rosehips, peppermint, nettles, hawthorn, goldenseal, fenugreek, cumin, capsicum, cinnamon, and basil.

It is a safe bet that eating a living-foods diet will provide an abundant supply from among the fifteen hundred known antioxidants that will help keep your body armed against the free radicals and therefore strong against disease.

A SELF-HEALING ORGANISM

The body is self-healing. Naturally, the greater the disease, the more effort must be put into the recovery process. But—unless the body has been brought to the edge of death through neglect or invasive medical intervention—it is always possible to reverse illness through the Hippocrates Health Program.

4

Sometimes It Really Is All in the Mind: A Program for Mental Health

Mental illness always has a physical component. It's also true that physical disease always has a mental component. A growing awareness of the mind/body connection has spawned reams of scientific research showing the tenacious relationship between physical and mental health. But many still remain skeptical, preferring to believe that the physical body is an entity entirely separate from the feelings and thoughts that drive our emotional and mental health.

THE PHYSICAL BASE OF MENTAL ILLNESS

I have seen psychological problems such as depression, paranoia, schizophrenia, and manic-depression disappear when psychological therapy was combined with a living-foods diet. Certainly, seeing is believing for me, but for you this may seem far-fetched. Yet, it should not be so hard to imagine that what we put into our body affects the way our mind works. Surely we see the connection between mental functioning and a popular drug called Prozac. Every day millions of people around the world contribute to a multimillion dollar industry by "eating" pills to treat their psychological disorders. It's only a small step further to recognize that other chemicals we ingest through food (pesticides, hormones, and additives) can cause the brain to react. On the positive side, nutrients, oxygen, and enzymes in living foods can nourish the brain and help treat malfunction.

Consider aberrant sexual behavior. Convicted sex offenders are sentenced to attend counseling programs that dig for the psychological root of the urges that lead to rape, pedophilia, and molestation. Ignored is the fact that these crimes often have a physical basis rather than, or along with, a psychological one. The problem can be hormonal and hormones can be affected by diet. Meat-eaters consume animal flesh that has been pumped full of hormones. Growth hormones are routinely used to fatten cattle. This meat also can be full of the hormone adrenaline that rushes through the animals in their last frantic moments before slaughter. When meat is eaten, these animal hormones create a hormonal imbalance in the human body, causing the body and mind to be overwhelmed with tension, confusion, violence, and aggression. Those with a certain amount of self-discipline and control are able—with a great deal of stress—to regulate these feelings. Those who lack self-control may constitute the sex offenders. Eliminate the cause, and the effects will be dramatically reduced. British prisons offer whole grains and vegetables to their inmates because they have found that this plant-based diet reduces the violence within the institutions. As an added benefit, it also helps reset the body's natural hormonal balance.

The *physical* effects of increased hormone consumption are easier to see and document—a number of studies have found that there has been a change in the average age of menstrual onset from age 12½ twenty years ago to about 9½ today. Many agree that this physical change may be the result of ingesting hormone-filled foods. It is my firm belief that a lot of sexual perversions, and many other forms of mental illness are also caused by an increase in the use of growth hormones in cattle, passed on via the high meat consumption in our society.

Although an extreme case, sexual deviates' consumption patterns do highlight the dramatic impact of diet on mental health.

Over the years, we have found that without exception the emotional obstructions of mental illness can be greatly exacerbated by 1) hormonal imbalances caused by eating meat products pumped full of hormones, 2) pesticide poisoning caused by ingesting pesticide residues on produce, and/or 3) a high body acidity level caused by eating animal and processed products. Living-foods vegetarians avoid the buildup of all these pollutants and increase the odds of mental health and activity throughout long lives.

DEPRESSION

A common mind/body relationship is seen in cases of depression. Depression results from three primary sources: poor self-image, lack of certain minerals needed by the nervous system, a hormonal imbalance that weakens the immune system. Although conventional medicine categorizes depression by the degree of emotional turmoil, the other two sources also play crucial roles. Depression is rare in individuals who have strong immune and nervous systems.

George Sweeten, age forty-five, came to the institute diagnosed with manic-depression. He had been on medication for this condition for many years but still suffered occasional bouts of mental instability. Our initial analysis of George's blood and urine found excess uric acid and an overall mineral imbalance in his body. We felt that the cause of the mental instability probably lay in George's monolithic diet—eating the same few foods every day and a reliance on animal products.

After two weeks on a living-foods diet, George noticed significant, positive changes in his personality. After one month, he chose to take himself off his medication. For the last ten years, George has been a living-foods vegetarian. He has been fully functioning without his medication or bouts of manic-depression.

George is just one of the hundreds of living testimonials to the effect of diet on depression.

ALCOHOLISM

Alcoholism is a perfect example of the interconnection between mental and physical needs. Hundreds of thousands of alcoholics around the world attend weekly counseling sessions trying to find the cause of their addiction. Because a shallow ego and low self-esteem are often characteristics of an alcoholic, psychological therapy and group support sessions are indeed helpful. However, ignoring the physical factors makes it very difficult to resist the craving for alcohol.

All alcoholics have either low or high blood-sugar levels, causing them to crave sugar. If you analyze plain white sugar and the sugar in alcohol, you'll find they are the same. When blood sugar drops, the alcohol pacifies the need. If you saturate the body with enough alcohol sugar, you effectively cross-circuit the brain—causing the equivalent of a psychological disorder. But the physical need for alcohol is at least as powerful as the psychological.

When alcoholics swear off the booze, they find they crave sweets and carbohydrates. They eat donuts, raisins, and chocolate bars. The sugar and the grain ferment in the digestive tract into alcohol within thirty to sixty minutes after eating and the craving is satisfied.

The alcoholic needs to be weaned off sugar with a living-foods diet. Once this is accomplished, the craving for alcohol is drastically diminished.

MEDICATION AND MENTAL ILLNESS

We do not advise anyone to give up prescribed medication; that is a personal decision one makes after a careful look at long-term physical and emotional needs. However, I can tell you that those who come to the institute and choose to stay on their medication almost always report that their physicians were subsequently happy to reduce the dosage based on their improved state. Those who choose to give up their medication completely often find that their diet and attitude changes expedite their recovery with greater comfort and speed than their medication was able to do.

Not only can medication sometimes slow recovery, it can actually *cause* the problem. I have even seen individuals diagnosed with physical and/or mental ailments that were later found to be caused by a mixture of prescribed medications. One case I remember in particular was that of a fellow named John Kavinn who was on daily medication for arthritis and heart disease. He took his medication faithfully for several years. Eventually, his mental faculties began to fail: his memory was weak and he had difficulty keeping his balance. Soon he was diagnosed with Alzheimer's disease. John came to the institute in hopes of improving his rapidly deteriorating physical and mental health.

John's physical health did dramatically improve on the Hippocrates Program, so he asked his physician to gradually reduce the dosage of his pills. As a result, the amount of medication coursing through the blood to his brain was reduced; at the same time, John's "mental infirmity" disappeared! Just as some drugs are "believed" to have a positive influence on mental illness, (valium and lithium, for example), it makes sense that others, or a combination of others, may have a negative effect.

THE MIND/BODY CONNECTION

In the same way that the physical condition of the nervous and immune systems can influence the quality of mental health, the state of your mental health can directly affect you physical well-being. Many dispute this, believing that the body functions independently of the mind. But to the contrary, the human mind exerts a powerful influence on even the most minute of cells. Today, stress-related illnesses such as hypertension, heart disease, and ulcers, will kill many more people than cancer. Others such as asthma, obesity, bad posture, tension, and dietary problems will cause chronic debilitating illnesses.

Taken together, these facts present us with the disturbing premise that even though we may observe every detail of the perfect diet, our mind can block good results. It is becoming more and more evident that our thinking must be positively channeled to get the full benefit of a sound, nutritional diet.

While a certain level of stress can be positive, prolonged and excessive levels are dangerous. Consistently high levels of stress have been directly linked to digestive disorders, chronic fatigue, anxiety, migraine headaches, and emotional disorders such as bulimia and anorexia. Test results indisputably have shown that the more major life changes you experience—for example, the death of a family member, divorce, changing jobs, or moving—the higher the risk of illness. It's also noteworthy that other factors such as coping style, social support system, and perception of the stress can strengthen or weaken a physical state.

In the classic research in this area, O. Carl Simonton found that cancer patients give up when faced with stress. Therefore, he concluded, cancer patients need to learn tenacity in fighting the disease and to be hopeful about the future. This, he felt, is facilitated by teaching cancer patients to deal with their social and emotional problems.[1] Additional research has shown that coping therapies can increase the disease-fighting cells called lymphocytes. We have recently discovered that happy thoughts increase the immune builders interferon, interluken, and imipramin, whereas unhappy thoughts produce the immune destroyers cortisol and adrenalin.

Other studies have found similar results. Researchers know that the ability to express anger appropriately is associated with increased survival and ability to cope with cancer. The following common themes are frequently found in the background history of cancer patients: loss of significant relationships prior to onset of tumor, inability to express hostile feelings, unresolved tension concerning parent figure, and feelings of hopelessness and helplessness.

Researchers have also found that not only can mental health trigger the onset of disease, it can affect the body's recuperative powers as well. Emotional turmoil, depression, grief, remorse, resentment, and other similar negative mental conditions have been found to severely restrict the regenerative capacity of the body.

We are only beginning to understand how and why mental outlook and physical health are connected. A theory proposed in 1995 suggests that tension triggers high levels of a hormone that helps germs and possibly even cancer cells to flourish. "If confirmed, this hypothesis would provide a direct link between the stress-related hormone and disease outcome," concluded Dr. Julio Licinio, one of the authors at the National Institute of Mental Health.[2]

SPONTANEOUS REMISSION

Researchers are also beginning to examine the way optimistic and positive thoughts *strengthen* the immune system. Since the thirteenth century, the sick and infirm have made pilgrimages to France hoping for a "miracle" at the fountain of Our Lady Of Lourdes. More than six thousand persons have claimed cures since 1858. Is it divine intervention or spontaneous remission generated by high hopes that returns physical health to these people?

Doctors use the terms *spontaneous regression* or *spontaneous remission* to describe an unexpected reversal of disease. Although not a common occurrence, cases of "miraculous" healing for which there is no medical explanation have been recorded all over the globe. Researchers continue to gather evidence that the mind plays an essential role in the physical processes that accompany remission. Recently the Institute of Noetic Sciences collected more than 3,500 accounts of spontaneous remission from 830 medical journals in more than twenty languages. Excerpts from these reports were published in 1993 by the Institute in *Spontaneous Remission—An Annotated Bibliography*. The stories are astounding, but true. They beg the question: "How can we doubt that one's attitude influences the outcome of disease?"

THE PLACEBO EFFECT

Western medicine calls substances that have suggestive effects, *place-bos,* from the Latin word *placere,* "to please." Research on placebos has shown that the effectiveness of even the most proven methodologies may be increased by what has been called the placebo halo—the expectation that the drugs will help. A case in the mid-1950s, in particular, illustrates the power of the placebo effect.

A Mr. Wright (a pseudonym) was a patient of Dr. Philip West and Dr. Bruno Klopfer. Wright was near death when he heard that a new cancer drug, Krebiozen, would soon be available for trial. Tumors the size of oranges were in Wright's neck, under his arms, and in his groin, chest, and abdomen. He burned with fever and required oxygen. His physicians believed he was "in a terminal state, untreatable, other than to give him sedatives to ease him on his way."

Wright received his first dose of Krebiozen on a Friday and became so sick that Dr. West believed that this first dose might be the last. But on Monday morning, West found the patient "walking around the ward, chatting happily with the nurses, and spreading his message of good cheer to anyone who would listen . . . The tumor masses had melted away like snowballs on a hot stove, and in only these few days, they were half their original size." When Wright's doctors discharged him from the hospital ten days later, the disease had all but vanished. Wright's story, however, was far from over.

Soon there was troubling news about Krebiozen. Very few patients improved, and newspapers were announcing that the "wonder drug" might be a failure. Wright followed this publicity grimly, and after two months of good health, gradually relapsed.

Dr. West decided to experiment. He reassured Wright that the newspapers were wrong, that Krebiozen was as promising as ever, and that the relapse was due only to a decline in the drug's potency. Deliberately playing on his patient's optimism, West promised that a shipment of "super-refined, double-strength" Krebiozen was on the way. "By delaying a couple of days before the 'shipment' arrived,"

West wrote, "his anticipation of salvation had reached a tremendous pitch. When I announced that the new series of injections were about to begin, he was almost ecstatic and his faith was very strong."

Wright's second recovery was even more dramatic than the first—although this time he was injected with nothing more than sterile water. Once again the tumors diminished, and soon the patient was "the picture of health." And so he remained, until the American Medical Association came forward with a formal announcement: "Nationwide tests show Krebiozen to be a worthless drug for the treatment of cancer." Within days, a dejected Wright checked into a hospital and quickly died.[3]

This case illustrates why the placebo response is a two-edged sword: it not only heals but kills.

PSYCHONEUROIMMUNOLOGY

The new science of psychoneuroimmunology (PNI) is zeroing in on the relationship between thoughts and feelings (which are expressed through our neurological anatomy—the brain and nervous system) and our immune system (which determines the state of our overall health). Let's take a look at the link-up points between our brain, nervous system, and immune system.

Connecting Links

New research shows that every thought and feeling we have generates measurable chemical and electrical changes in our brain and through-out the body. Emotional response, which is present to some degree with every experience, tends to be concentrated within the limbic system in the central area of the brain, where the hypothalamus resides. This emotional information is actually transferred from the limbic system to receptor sites that act like satellite dishes in our endocrine glands (pituitary, thalamus, pancreas, adrenals) receiving signals from biologically encoded neuropeptides, or chains of complex amino acids.

Interestingly enough, key components of the immune system called monocytes have receptor sites for these same neuropeptides! There is important research indicating that nerve tissue running through every major organ of the body links the immune system to the central nervous system via these monocytes. It seems that monocytes link the emotional responses in the brain directly to the immune system.

In test-tube experiments over the years, scientists had watched immune cells attack foreign bacteria without help from either body or mind. The immune system seemed completely autonomous, able to fight disease on its own. But now we understand that the immune system is not an independent defender against disease; it is a team player. What we had thought of as our primary defense system is in fact only one part of a complex, interactive, mind/body network. The new science of psychoneuroimmunology (which has been used at the institute successfully for many years) shows that the brain, nervous system, and immune system are cooperative parts of a larger system that reacts to stress.

A Mind/Body Model

Herpes viruses offer a helpful model for studying the effects of stress on immunity: the viruses are very common, and unlike other viruses, herpes viruses are never completely wiped out by the immune system but simply are held in check by immune response. Diseases caused by herpes viruses often come and go as the virus advances and retreats. Specific herpes viruses are responsible for recurring oral cold sores and genital ulcers, as well as for chicken pox and for its recurring form, known as shingles.

The activity of herpes viruses in the body provides a rough measure of the effectiveness of the immune system in holding them back. Researchers can judge this reaction by measuring antibodies to the virus in a person's blood. Having more herpes antibodies, or lower immunity, has been associated with many kinds of stress. Students showed more herpes antibodies while undergoing exams than they did after summer vacation[4], and divorced and separated men and women showed more antibodies than a matched group of married persons.[5]

The same association between stress and herpes holds true for the actual occurrence of disease. In one study, researchers from the University of Pennsylvania and Veterans Administration Hospital in Philadelphia found that typically unhappy people experienced more cold sores than happier subjects.[6] In another study, psychologist Margaret Kemeny found that among a group of thirty-six people suffering from the genital form of herpes, depressed individuals experienced more frequent recurrence of the disease.[7]

This research provides strong evidence once more that micro-organisms alone do not cause infectious disease—that the emotional condition of the person exposed to the microorganism also matters. In the more than forty years since the earliest experiments on stress and immune function, we have moved from the belief that the immune system acts independently of the brain, to the belief that the immune system may be influenced by the brain, to a new idea entirely: that the brain and the immune system may be part of an integrated system, working together for the body's health.

BUILDING MENTAL HEALTH

Just as we are what we eat, we are what we think and feel. Just as we must assimilate our food and keep our physical bodies clean, we equally must integrate feelings and unfetter our emotional expression if we are to attain total health. As part of the Hippocrates Health Program, we encourage all our guests to develop the habit of building strong mental health through relaxation therapies. These include laughter, guided visual imagery, deep breathing, meditation, prayer, and biofeedback.

RELAXATION THERAPIES

Relaxation doesn't mean bed rest. Relaxation techniques involve various self-help strategies to control the involuntary workings of the nervous system such as blood pressure, heart rate, respiration, and metabolism. In addition to their effect on these bodily functions, relaxation techniques can decrease muscle tension, relieve anxiety, and encourage restful sleep.

The roots of our physical response to stress go back to primitive days. In those times, the difference between fighting off an animal and being eaten by the animal lay in a person's ability to react quickly to danger. The human body had to be able to prepare for fight or flight at a moment's notice. To do this, breathing became faster and shallower to bring more oxygen into the body quickly. The heartbeat increased to push that oxygen through the bloodstream rapidly. And the blood flow was redirected from the internal organs and surface of the body to the deep muscles, which needed more energy to prepare for a fight or flight. The people who had quick stress-response systems survived.

The problem is that this stress response, which was designed for life-or-death combat and escape, is no longer appropriate for us. Today, we typically don't need extra oxygen directed to our deep muscles when we feel stress or pain, yet it still happens. Our body prepares us to fight or flee, but most often we have no visible foe. So what happens? Our heart beats rapidly, our blood pressure becomes elevated, our muscles tighten—all with no release. After a while, our body begins to wear down. We develop physical problems such as ulcers, headaches, heart palpitations, backaches, rashes, colitis, allergies, asthma, heart disease, diabetes, chronic pain syndromes, and even cancer.

Stress contributes to the intensity, frequency, and duration of disease and pain. But we also know that stress is a treatable condition that can be controlled with relaxation therapies. These techniques influence general health, disease, pain, and chronic illnesses in several ways:

1. Self-regulated stress management improves your sense of control over your health. Cognitive therapists assure us that the way we think about our health does affect it. Relaxation techniques put you in charge; they give you an active role in managing your health. This alone reduces the feelings of helplessness and hopelessness that support and maintain illness.
2. Relaxation techniques reduce anxiety. It's difficult to think positively if you are chronically anxious and tense. Relaxation techniques give you a sense of ease and determination.
3. Relaxation enriches sleep; anxiety impoverishes it. Relaxation techniques calm the body, improve circulation, lower anxiety levels, and promote peaceful rest.
4. Relaxation techniques improve overall well-being. If a stress response is chronic, the constant presence of adrenaline in the body begins to wear down the immune system. Relaxation techniques help you achieve the psychological state that leads to a strong and healthy body.

Most relaxation techniques can be practiced anywhere at your convenience without special apparatus or devices. But to learn the strategies, it's best to practice them in a comfortable, quiet spot, free of distractions. Once certain techniques are learned, they can be pulled out whenever you feel stressed. They are available not only in times of emergency but to maintain a healthy and calm state of being. Of course, no one can completely eliminate the stress of daily living or the stress of pain and illness, but you can learn to manage it.

You'll need to experiment a bit to find out which of the following relaxation techniques work best for you. Some take effort and practice, so don't give up too soon on any one. Try them all; give each one a chance to prove its worth. Then choose a few that you feel comfortable doing. Relaxation therapy is a lifelong skill that will improve the quality of your life, health, and well-being.

Laughter

Ever since Norman Cousins wrote his best-selling book, *Anatomy of an Illness*, in which he described how he conquered a degenerative illness through a steady diet of laughter, there has been a growing interest in laughter therapy as a curative. Even staunch doubters are gradually accepting this idea in light of the growing store of research evidence.

At the DeKalb General Hospital in Decatur, Georgia, a "humor room" was established that contains no medical equipment at all. Doctors order their discouraged and listless patients to visit this room regularly as an important adjunct to other treatment.

The cheerful, brightly-lit room contains a large video library of old television comedy shows and old movies featuring Charlie Chaplin, Laurel and Hardy, Buster Keaton, W. C. Fields, Red Skelton, the Marx Brothers, Abbott and Costello, and other comics.

Some results have been truly remarkable—most have been encouraging. Nurses have noticed that after spending only a couple of hours a day in this room, patients usually perk up and have a rekindled desire to become well and return home.

Patients in other hospitals in Orlando, Schenectady, Houston, Phoenix, Los Angeles, Stockholm, and London are also being offered laughter therapy. Some hospitals have found that group humor sessions comprising joke telling, humorous anecdotes, recitation of comic plays, and skit presentations are enhanced by the positive energy of a social dynamic.

Besides these social and psychological benefits, research reveals that there are many physiological benefits that are derived from laughter sessions. Blood pressure is reduced and the cardiovascular system is stimulated. Also, muscular tension is reduced, and the respiratory system receives a beneficial increase of oxygen.

Laughter also affects the production of endorphins, which are the body's natural pain killers. It seems that the eighty facial muscles involved in laughing affect the cranial blood flow and alter brain temperature which, in turn, influences the synthesis of endorphins. Also, there are indications that laughter may stimulate the thymus gland, which helps the body to withstand disease.

Family members who care for sick relatives are also very good candidates for this therapy. These caregivers are particularly vulnerable to fatigue and anxiety, which may result in unacceptable stress levels. Both the patient and the caregiver can benefit from daily humor sessions. Norman Cousins reported that five minutes of intense positive thinking, such as laughter, can cause a 53 percent increase in the disease-fighting ability of blood. Even a few minutes of laughter has been found to result in hours of relaxation. Starting today, find something to laugh about.

Guided Visual Imagery

Because we all daydream and nightdream, we know we have an internal world that we can experience in both positive and negative ways. Guided imagery requires you to go to that inner world and construct a place where you'll feel safe and relaxed whenever you imagine yourself being there. The core of the guided imagery approach to stress reduction lies in imagining a positive experience in order to stop, interrupt, or prevent a physical stress reaction.

To do this, create a positive image in your mind that represents a safe and relaxing environment. Practice visiting this imaginary place over and over again. Then, when you're stressed, you can go there just briefly and benefit from the relaxed feeling it gives you. For example, you may find this image soothing:

> *I am stretched out on an ocean beach. The sun is warm on my body. When it gets too strong, I have an umbrella for protection. I feel the warmth of the sand on my fingertips. I see the calm ocean touching the shore. I can smell the salt of the ocean, and I can taste the sea air. On my beach, are just the right number of people—I'm not crowded or lonely. No sand crabs crawl, no flies swarm. I feel*

just wonderful. It's an ideal place that I can visit with all my senses anytime I want. Even when I'm in the middle of a crowd with my eyes wide open, I can go to my beach.

This safe place happens to be a beach—yours can be anywhere. It can be in your family room by the fireplace, the woods by a stream, the park down the street. But keep these points in mind:

- Make the place real. When you're stressed or in pain, you won't be able to relate to an alien planet.
- Involve all of your senses. Pick smells, touches, tastes, sounds, and sights that are pleasing to you.
- Go to this place often. The more you practice increasing the vividness of your image, the more you can rely on it when you feel stressed.

Another kind of guided imagery is sometimes used to battle chronic disease and pain under the guidance of a trained therapist. Introduced in the 1970s to help athletes and musicians perform better, the method has won increasing acceptance as a medical tool. Patients are taught how their immune system is affected by their disease, pain, and stress. Then with cues from the therapist or a tape recording, they learn to visualize their condition and "see" the body fighting against the disease and restoring comfort and health. A person suffering from the pain of arthritis in the hands, for example, might mentally see her inflamed and stiff joints regain flexible, fluid movement. This mental picture temporarily can dissuade the brain from transmitting pain.

Deep Breathing

Because the body needs oxygen to fuel its stress response, you can reduce or short-circuit the stress you feel by regaining control of your breathing. Athletes often do this just before a race begins or as they are about to get up to bat.

Follow these instructions to stop the shallow, rapid breathing that accompanies a stress response:

- Put your hand on your stomach.
- Take a deep breath from the bottom of your stomach.
- Breathe in as you silently count to five.
- Feel it fill you with warm air.
- Feel your hand rise with your stomach muscles.
- Exhale. Don't push it out. Let it release gently to the count of five.
- When you let out the air, smile.
- Do this sequence twice.
- Then breathe regularly (rhythmically and comfortably).
- Breathe deeply again after you have let a minute or two go by.
- Repeat this deep-breathing/regular breathing cycle two or three times, or more if needed, until you find your breathing has returned to a natural, comfortable pace.

It's recommended that you smile when you exhale because smiling is a natural mood elevator. While you're smiling, it's difficult to be stressed. Try this experiment: Think nasty thoughts while you're smiling. Isn't it hard?

Deep breathing is a relaxation technique you can use anywhere. No one around needs to know you're practicing stress-reduction. Use it whenever you feel your body tensing from stress.

Meditation

Meditation can be used to enhance the effectiveness of deep breathing. Deep breathing can arrest a stress response, but too often the effort is sabotaged by the appearance of negative thoughts. Meditation can counter the intrusion of this renewed stress.

Meditation helps you focus on in the present moment in a state called mindfulness. The process heals not only physically, but emotionally as well. The physical benefits come from the relaxation response, the tuning down of the body's stress. Emotionally, meditation decreases anxiety and calms the mind.

In the early 1970s, the proponents of transcendental meditation, or TM, wanted to scientifically measure their practice. They asked Harvard cardiologist Herbert Benson and another researcher, R. Keith Wallace, to monitor meditators for physiological change. The scientists wired the subjects with electrodes and drew blood samples before and after meditation. What they discovered confirmed that the calm felt by TM practitioners was definitely not "all in their minds" but a unique physiological state distinct from either simple rest or sleep. It was as if the fight-or-flight response shifted into reverse. Heart and breathing rates and blood pressure went down, and so did the rate at which meditators consumed oxygen. Moreover, this physiological calm occurred within minutes. TM seemed like an ever-ready antidote to the health-eroding stress of modern life.[8]

Dr. Benson went on to strip meditation of its spiritual trappings. What was important, he suggested, was the act of quiet concentration. Benson termed the resulting physiological reaction "the relaxation response." This was also the title of his 1976 book, which became a best seller and a major influence on a generation of health practitioners.

Whether pursued simply for relaxation or for spiritual enlightenment or healing, meditation requires a quiet, comfortable setting as well as a conscious effort to relax the muscles, regulate the breathing, and calm the mind. A point of focus is needed: You can use a special word, called a mantra or focal point; this can be the word "calm" or "peace" or even a meaningless sound. Or you can direct your mind toward a calming mental image, or to the simple rhythm of your own breathing.

Many programs of meditation are available, but for a sample of a basic meditative style, follow these instructions:

Sit comfortably in a quiet place, free of distractions. Close your eyes and breathe freely for a few seconds to focus your mind on relaxation. Then to begin your meditation, exhale a deep breath, and focus on your mantra; say this word silently to yourself. As you breathe in, your mind may still have a stressful thought, but as you breathe out, switch your attention back to your mantra. Do this for about fifteen to thirty minutes. With practice, you'll be able to breathe and meditate without stressful thoughts bothering you. This stress-free, relaxed time will give your body opportunity to rejuvenate and calm itself.

Prayer

The healing power of prayer has been claimed by every religion in recorded history. To this day, millions of people find religious prayer to be comforting, relaxing, and a source of inner strength. But the mind/body connections between prayer and healing are now being scientifically studied. Dr. Larry Dossey, author of *Healing Words: The Power of Prayer and the Practice of Medicine,* has researched the healing effect of praying: both by praying oneself and being prayed for by others. Time and time again, he has shown that the immune system strengthens after prayer. It has also been found that the effect even can be transmitted from one to another over thousands of miles. As of 1996, at least ten different universities in North America were studying the power of prayer.

Like meditation, prayer is a time for tuning out the outer world and focusing on an internal life that can dictate the course of health.

Biofeedback

Biofeedback gives you concrete evidence of the mind's influence on the body's functions. In a healthy person, physiological functions are performed and regulated by the brain and central nervous system. The mind, however, often interferes when under stress, which produces tension in the body. Biofeedback can teach you to intervene to restore balanced functioning in the body.

Conscious control of your stress level can affect many body functions that can be accurately and continuously measured, such as heart rate, skin temperature, blood pressure, muscle tension, and brain waves. The biofeedback equipment that measures these functions includes the electroencephalograph (EEG), which records nerve and brain waves; the electromyograph (EMG), which registers muscle tension; and the galvanic skin resistance instrument (GSR), which detects the electrical conductivity of the skin to record states of arousal, excitement, or nervousness.

When they are hooked up to subjects, these machines convey information through signals that can be easily interpreted. For instance, when the instrument detects muscle tension, a red light might go on or a certain sound might be emitted to signal what is happening to you internally. You would then begin certain relaxation techniques to control muscle tension. The techniques that are used in combination with the biofeedback equipment include relaxation and autosuggestion exercises, visual imagery, and meditation and prayer. For example, if the equipment signals that your heart rate is increasing, you can slow the heart beat by imagining a calm, peaceful place where you feel relaxed and safe.

Biofeedback has many applications. It is used as an effective treatment for emotional or behavioral problems, such as anxiety, depression, phobias, insomnia, and tension headaches. It also can be used to treat illnesses considered by some professionals to be psychosomatic, such as asthma, ulcers, colitis, diarrhea, cardiac arrhythmia, hypertension, Raynaud's syndrome, and migraines. Biofeedback can help people with neuromuscular problems caused by stroke or cerebral palsy. Because biofeedback increases your understanding of your total mind/body functioning, it also can be beneficial in enhancing personal growth and awareness.

It is best to undergo biofeedback treatments under the supervision of a psychologist trained in biofeedback.

THE MIND/BODY CONNECTION

Skepticism of the mind/body connection is gradually eroding in the face of scientific evidence. Research is showing, for example, that breast cancer patients who receive group support may live, on average, twice as long as those who do not. Other experiments have revealed that hypnosis can hasten the healing of burns, that laughter can increase immune function, and that diabetics can lower their need for insulin with relaxation techniques. Psychologists have sketched out personality types associated with heart disease, and studies linking psychological factors to illness and immune function now number in the thousands. This does not, of course, prove that humans can heal themselves of cancer or other diseases. Nor does it prove that illness is "all in the head" or that we cause our own sickness. What the studies do suggest, however, is that feelings and emotions influence health, and that the body's healing system may be far more powerful and complex than we have dared imagine. An ever-growing body of evidence shows that thoughts, feelings, and attitudes can push us toward illness or toward health.

5

Counting Food Energy: Living Foods and Weight Management

Guests at the institute often ask, "Will I lose weight on the Hippocrates diet?" Some want to lose extra pounds; others worry that they'll lose more than they want or need to. The surprising truth is this: the Hippocrates diet can meet the needs of those who are overweight, underweight, and normal weight. The nourishment of living foods fuels the body with the energy needed to maintain optimal health and body size—no more, no less. So if you are overweight, you will lose all your excess weight on this program. If you are slender, you will maintain the weight and body size you now have. If you are underweight, the Hippocrates Health Program can help you put on the additional pounds you need in order to achieve robust health.

WEIGHT LOSS IN THE PAST

Let's take a quick look at our fascination with dieting during this century:

- Before 1917, the word "calorie" was used only in physics and was introduced to the common vocabulary by Lulu Hunt Peters, publisher of the popular food magazine *Diet and Health*.
- In 1939, "miracle" diet pills generated sales of $30 million annually until the FDA stepped in.
- In 1943, the Metropolitan Life insurance company published the first ideal weight tables for women.
- In 1959, the *New York Times* reported that Americans suffered from a "dieting neurosis."
- In 1967, the fashion model Twiggy, 5'7" and 91 pounds, appeared on the cover of *Vogue* four times.
- In the 1970s, the Atkins, Scarsdale, Stillman, and Pritikin diets turned our attention to diets recommended by physicians and based on theories of good nutrition.
- In 1982, Johns Hopkins University researchers calculated that Americans had bought into 29,068 "theories, treatments, and outright schemes to lose weight."
- In 1990, television talk show host Oprah Winfrey brought her weight battle into our living rooms and lost sixty-seven pounds on her Optifast liquid protein diet.

It's been a long road to the Hippocrates diet. Now with objective distance, we can more easily see what was hype, what was dangerous, and why most weight-loss diets were ultimately dismal failures.

Starving Our Way to Good Looks

Ordinary slimming diets are notoriously poor nutritionally. The grapefruit diet, fasting diets, and the thousands of "Seven-Day Diets" heralded from the covers of women's magazines starve the body of more than just calories and fat. They restrict the very life-giving fuel the human body needs to function.

Because these diets are short on vitamins, minerals, and other essential nutrients, the body (in desperate bid for nutritional satisfaction) demands more and more calories. So when starvation can no longer be ignored and the diet is discarded, the dieter overeats. This bingeing on non-nutritional foods produces poisonous wastes that the body can't get rid of. As a survival technique, the body stores the excess waste in the layer of fat under the skin. The body's need for more energy than most slimming diets provide triggers bingeing, bad eating habits, and more weight gain.

Fasting is another popular but dangerous and counterproductive weight-loss strategy. Without a steady supply of glucose from carbohydrates, the body turns to its own protein and fat to meet its energy needs. Protein is borrowed from tissues, muscles, and organs, converted into glucose, and burned for fuel. By the end of a long fast, huge amounts of protein along with smaller quantities of fat, have been used by the body for energy. The result can be a total weakening of the organs and body tissues—damage that may take years to rebuild, and even then only if the maintenance diet used is adequate in carbohydrates for energy and in vitamins, minerals, proteins, and enzymes for assimilation. Adding insult to injury, the body is more prone to weight gain after a fast due to its weakened condition.

Merely counting calories is another sure way to sabotage a diet because reducing or increasing calories alone results in a faulty system of weight management. It is not the calories in a food that wholly determine if the body will store it as fat. In many cases, nutritious foods have a higher caloric value than junk foods, but only the nutritious foods (being rich in enzymes, oxygen, trace minerals, and nutrients) are going to be absorbed and utilized by the body without causing weight gain. The lower-calorie piece of junk food is not absorbed or easily eliminated and it remains in the body as stored fat. Because calories are not the focus of healthy weight maintenance, you'll note that in this chapter, the Hippocrates Program does not use the word "calorie" but rather uses the word "energy." This more aptly describes what we gain from our food.

"Healthy" Diets That Went Wrong

The Atkins, Scarsdale, and Stillman diets of the 1970s put a new spin on weight reduction. They were formulated by medical physicians and supposedly based on the nutritional needs of the body. Hundreds of thousands of people bought their books, went to their workshops, and contributed much time and effort to these weight-loss programs. Still, most failed in the long run.

In 1972, *Dr. Atkins' Diet Revolution* hit the bookstores with great acclaim. The diet guaranteed weight loss by counteracting the metabolic imbalance that causes people to get fat in the first place. It's true that metabolic imbalances contribute to weight gain, but Atkins tried to find a balance by cutting out carbohydrates. (As we now know, carbohydrates promote weight loss by burning efficiently and cleanly, breaking down to safe water and carbon dioxide.) He also ignored (or did not at that time fully understand) the destructive potential of high-fat foods. Happy to assure dieters that they could lose weight without counting calories, Atkins bragged that others who followed his diet had "lost weight on bacon and eggs for breakfast, on heavy cream in their coffee, on mayonnaise in their salads, butter sauce on their lobster, on spareribs, roast duck, and pastrami."[1] Exactly where did Atkins expect the excess fat from this kind of diet to go? Disillusioned dieters found that it was stored in their bodies.

In 1974, *Dr. Stillman's 14-Day Shape Up Program* was published.[2] This popular book advocated the combination of diet and exercise for weight loss. This was a sound and proven idea, but Stillman's guarantee of a "miracle" weight loss of twenty-five pounds or more in just fourteen days on his Protein-PLUS diet (high protein low-carbohydrate) and just ten minutes of exercise a day was too good to be true. Stillman assured readers that they could return to their normal diet after the fourteen-day program. Yes, the weight dropped off on this diet, which was 80 percent to 90 percent protein and only

5 percent carbohydrate and 5 percent fat. But that kind of weight loss can be sustained for no more than fourteen days; the diet's end brought a quick return of any lost weight.

In 1978, *The Complete Scarsdale Medical Diet* was written by Dr. Herman Tarnower. This highly restrictive diet reduced carbohydrate consumption to 34.5 percent of daily intake (with protein up at 43 percent) and put great emphasis on calorie counting. Dieters were limited to one thousand calories a day and strict adherence to a detailed daily menu with the warning, "Eat exactly what is assigned. Don't substitute."[3] Tarnower may not have fully understood the psychology of deprivation that sabotages any diet, but he should have known that any man or woman, whether active or inactive, needs more than a thousand calories a day to survive without extreme fatigue and eventual malnourishment. Again, thousands of dieters struggled through the program feeling tired, light-headed, and generally ill and tried to ignore the body's cry for fuel.

The Atkins, Stillman, and Scarsdale diets all boasted that they caused increased body-fat metabolism and the production of ketones. Ketones are the waste products of partially burned (or metabolized) fat. "If you are producing ketones," stated Tarnower, "it is a sign that your body is burning off fat at an accelerated rate; you are enjoying *Fast Fat Metabolism*. And this is what we want."[4] Apparently, Atkins, Tarnower, and Stillman did not know how dangerous ketones can be. Being acidic, they can change the nearly neutral pH of the blood. We've already seen in chapter 3 what happens to the health of the body when the blood levels turn acidic. In addition, a sudden change of diet can produce a rapid rise in the acid level, producing a diabetic-like state. The ultimate danger of excessive ketones is ketoacidosis, which can be fatal.

The Atkins, Scarsdale, and Stillman diets all recommended high-protein intake. This is the reason for the dramatic stories of successful weight loss. As the body attempts to dilute the toxic by-products of the excess protein ingested, large amounts of water are lost from the body tissues shortly after the diet is begun. Then weight is lost quickly with the elimination of the water and the toxins it carries out of the body. But a week or so into the diet, the dieter hits a plateau. When the diet is discontinued, the dieter gains weight rapidly. In Dr. Atkins' own words, "I concede that the worst feature about this diet is the rapidity with which you gain if you abandon it."[5]

Rapid weight gain is not really the worst feature. High-protein or liquid protein (like Oprah's Optifast) diets cause physical damage to the body. They might cause kidney damage through ketosis; might bring on gout; might increase cholesterol and triglyceride levels, stressing the heart; might damage the liver; might cause constipation due to the excessive use of fiber-poor animal foods; might wash minerals and vitamins out of the body, causing tiredness, bone damage, and tooth decay; and might increase the risk of certain types of cancer. It's now clear that not only do high-protein diets fail to keep weight off—they are dangerous.

A Victory in the Diet War

In 1979, Nathan Pritikin wrote *The Pritikin Program for Diet and Exercise*. This was the first diet system to make a declaration of war against processed foods, fats, sugars, proteins, salt, caffeine, and alcohol. Pritikin recommended a lowfat, low-protein, and high carbohydrate diet that restricted meat and fish to under a quarter pound daily. Pritikin declared, "Foods high in complex carbohydrates—grains, vegetables, and fruits—are the best foods you can eat."[6] He threw away the calorie counting and starvation that seemed synonymous with the word "diet." He offered medical proof that good health depended on appropriate body weight and sound nutritional diet plan. He also added exercise to the diet formula. Although Pritikin did not acknowledge that there is a psychological component to the reason why people overeat (in fact he ridiculed the idea), his work brought international attention to a high-carbohydrate weight-management program that legitimately promised weight loss and good health.

Why Lose Weight?

Nathan Pritikin brought us more than a new way of dieting; he gave us new reasons for losing weight. The vanity and social pressure that fueled the diets of earlier years were now nudged from the foreground by health concerns. Pritikin demonstrated that a healthy diet and appropriate body weight directly influenced one's health.

Today, we know that overweight people do not live as long as lean people, and they are a lot less healthy while they are alive. Obesity increases the risks of developing diabetes, heart disease, hypertension, arteriosclerosis, gall bladder disease, and certain types of cancer. It aggravates gouty arthritis, damages the liver, increases the risk of hernias, and causes difficulty in pregnancy and childbirth.

Putting more food into the body than is needed results in stress to the heart and blood vessels. Blood and lymph circulation slows and causes blood pressure to rise. If you are a man between the ages of thirty-five and fifty, your chance of developing heart disease increases by 30 percent for each ten pounds you gain above your ideal weight.

Obesity, defined as being more than 20 percent over ideal weight, causes twenty million new illnesses in the U.S. every year and kills 300,000 people. "We are literally in the midst of an obesity epidemic," says Judith Stern, vice president of the American Obesity Association. While thousands diet to drop their excess pounds, almost all of the few who succeed regain the weight within five years. No wonder so many have given up hope.

So Why Not?

The more we find reasons for maintaining an appropriate body weight, the more excuses emerge for not losing weight:

"I diet constantly, but I never lose any weight."

Excess weight is not caused by eating too much food. It's caused by eating the wrong foods. The typical diet we eat today is high in fat and low in carbohydrates. Processing has removed the low-calorie fiber and bulk from most foods. What is left is unbalanced, condensed, and fattening food that can't be absorbed or eliminated from the body. It is stored as fat deposits and can cause obesity.

"I have a medical problem that keeps me from losing weight."

Some say they have an underactive thyroid that causes their weight problem. The fact is, hypothyroidism as a cause of weight gain is rare and can be treated easily. Others argue that their pituitary gland fails to respond to the body's signals that hunger is abated, and so they continue to eat. In rare cases, this may be true. But for most of us, it probably is not.

"Fat runs in my family."

Some look to genetics for answers to their problem with excess weight. It's true that certain body types hold more weight, but that doesn't mean they can't become lean. Most people who have been fat since birth have a normal number of fat cells, but an abnormal amount of fat in them. A regulated metabolism (which can be developed through the Hippocrates Program) is the key to maintaining a healthy body weight.

MODERN SCIENCE AND FAT SUBSTITUTES

Modern science has found a way to let us keep our excuses and lose weight too. In 1996, Procter & Gamble received FDA approval for a fat substitute called Olestra. Olestra is a synthetic product made from sugar and fatty acids, and because it passes through the body without being absorbed, it has no calories. Olestra also has a property known as "mouth feel," which makes fat-free food seem rich and creamy. It has been approved for use in salted snacks such as chips, popcorn, and crackers, and other uses are expected in the near future.

The FDA acknowledges that Olestra is not without negative side-effects. Products containing Olestra must carry a warning label reading: "This product contains Olestra. Olestra may cause abdominal cramping. . . . Olestra inhibits the absorption of some vitamins and other nutrients. Vitamins A, D, E, and K have been added." If the whole truth be known, the warning label should be much longer. Dr. Sheldon Margen, a professor of public health at the University of California, Berkeley, and Dale A. Ogar, the managing editor of the university's *Wellness Letter* have reported these additional concerns in their syndicated column "Nutrition & You":

- Olestra can deplete the body of fat-soluble vitamins, including A, D, E, and K, as well as beta carotene and other important carotenoids. In one of Procter & Gamble's own studies, researchers found that eating sixteen Olestra potato chips a day for eight weeks reduced the level of carotenoids in the blood by 50 percent.
- Some animal studies found liver-cell changes that raise a suspicion about potential cancer risk.
- Diarrhea and cramping are known risks of eating Olestra. The physical properties of this fat substitute are similar to mineral oil, which is a well-known laxative. Long-term use of any laxative is unhealthful.[7]

The effort to create products that let us have our cake and eat it too cater to all the excuses we make for not watching our weight. But the fact remains that a truly healthful and fit lifestyle requires some effort and knowledge of what the body really needs to maintain its proper weight. The Hippocrates diet needs no warning label.

HIPPOCRATES WEIGHT MANAGEMENT

So, you're wondering, how does the Hippocrates Health Program fit into this emerging picture of diet plans? The answer is simple and straightforward: The Hippocrates Health Program is unbeatable for safe, effective, long-lasting weight loss, gain, or maintenance. It combines a healthful diet with exercise; it acknowledges the psychological factors involved in dieting, and comes up with a no-fail program.

For Weight Loss

The Hippocrates diet is high in carbohydrates, rich in vitamins and minerals, and low in fat—similar to the best working examples of modern weight loss plans (like the Pritikin diet). But the Hippocrates diet has a unique feature—enzymes. Enzymes break down the excess fat that needs to be eliminated in weight loss. An examination of the fat deposits of individuals weighing between three hundred pounds and five hundred pounds reveals decreased levels of fat-splitting lipase enzymes. Only enzymes do the work of breaking up fat deposits and eliminating them, so a diet void of enzyme-rich food (no matter how restrictive or low-calorie) is bound to frustrate dieters in the long run. Most diets, even the best ones, fail to get results because of the absence of enzymes in them. Cooked, enzymeless food is fattening; the same amounts of raw food are not.

The Hippocrates approach to dieting works with nature rather than against it. A living-foods diet does not mean starvation—it means supernutrition and slow, steady, healthy weight loss. You do not have to count calories or weigh out bird-size portions on kitchen scales or feel deprived when you do not eat and guilty when you do. The same living-foods diet that nourishes and heals those with diabetes and arthritis works wonders for the overweight.

The Hippocrates diet helps you lose weight by working with the body's natural digestive mechanisms to do the following:

1. Eliminate cravings by giving your body all the nutrients and calories it needs
2. Restore healthy functioning to the digestive system to gain maximum benefit from the foods you eat and eliminate the waste before it turns into fat
3. Supply the enzymes needed to break up and eliminate fat deposits

After a few weeks of eating living foods, you will naturally tend to eat less. You will feel more full on raw foods because they contain a lot of fiber and essential nutrients. Your body will not constantly cry out for more. Those awful cravings that lead to excessive eating and obesity belong to cooked diets.

The bottom line is this: The rate of obesity is rising because we eat too much high-calorie food without enzymes or fiber, and not enough uncooked, unprocessed whole fruits, vegetables, sprouts, beans, and grains. Processed foods are too dense in calories and provide little energy. It takes thirty ears of corn to make the oil needed to fry an average serving of French fries. Two pounds of beets are needed to produce the sugar that flavors the fruit pie and soft drink in a typical fast-food meal. These items, and other overrefined and concentrated foods, have less fiber to fill up space in your stomach than do foods in their whole state. You can eat more processed foods than whole foods (and get their extra calories) and still feel less full. If you balance lower and higher-energy whole living foods, you cannot fit enough food in your stomach in three satisfying meals to become obese! It's that simple.

Weight Loss Tips

At the institute, I have worked with thousands of overweight people, nearly all of whom have had immediate weight reductions on the Hippocrates diet. Most of the raw fruits and vegetables used in salads are fat-free foods and are rich sources of vitamins and minerals. A mistake some people make when they leave the institute is to eat plenty of fat-free salads, but then turn to cooked foods to get the bulk of their diet. For best results, the majority of the energy units in your diet should come from raw foods.

When trying to lose weight on the Hippocrates diet, high-energy raw foods such as sprouted beans, vegetables, sprouted grains, some fruits, and nuts (and recipes made from them) should be used each day. These foods are richly nourishing; they will fill you up, but not out. They will also supply you with plenty of energy.

These foods are also rich in enzymes, which guarantee efficient and total digestion. The food enzymes in the Hippocrates diet attack stores of fat and unwanted tissue, breaking them down cell by cell and eliminating them. Remember: only enzymes can do the work of breaking up fat cells and eliminating their waste. Living foods and juices require less of your digestive juices than cooked foods do. This allows your body's internal "house cleaning crew" to use all of its enzyme strength to break down and eliminate unwanted fat cells. In people eating cooked foods, this enzyme strength is tied up by the digestive system and is unable to help break down the excess fat unless they literally starve themselves. On the Hippocrates diet, you can eat living, fresh foods to your heart's content, and still lose weight safely and surely.

You can maximize your weight loss if you periodically eat mostly living foods that adjust your metabolism and are naturally low in calories—especially grain and bean sprouts, greens, and sliced vegetables in salads, with plenty of sprout juices. A week every month of this low-calorie diet will be often enough. But for the other three weeks of the month, follow the standard Hippocrates diet, using all the different foods and food groups, including those higher in energy units. The higher-calorie living foods will help you feel satisfied.

If you are overweight and stay physically active (see "Weight Loss and Exercise," page 103), you should easily drop one to three pounds a week if you stick to the diet. Don't try to lose weight too rapidly, though. Shedding pounds too quickly can lead to loss of muscle and body protein, dehydration, acidosis, menstrual troubles, back pains, and hypoglycemia (low blood sugar). Eat! For breakfast have watermelon juice or dilute one-third fruit juice to two-thirds water. If you need more, try grain cereal with rice milk. At lunch, eat a big salad with all kinds of sprouts and a seed, avocado, or vegetable dressing; a handful of sprouted almonds; or some bread with sprouted bean spread. For dinner, try soup, grain crisps, vegetable loaf, and occasionally, two hours after your meal, a piece of raw fruit pie. There's no need to make dieting a drag and starve yourself, when all it takes is a little creativity, time, and effort to really enjoy your new diet.

Weight Loss and Exercise

You can't rely on exercise alone to slough off extra pounds—if excess waste and cooked and processed foods continue to stream into the body, even the ardent exerciser will lose hardly any weight. But when combined with the Hippocrates diet, even light exercise will help shed pounds. A half hour or more of light exercise such as brisk walking also stimulates the secretion of epinephrine, or adrenaline, which helps to suppress the appetite. Conversely, activity below a certain level can increase the appetite, so the "right amount" of exercise certainly belongs in your weight-loss program.

We used to think that high-impact aerobic exercises were the best kind of exercise for weight loss. But we now understand that the jolt of these exercises to the skeletal structure is very stressful and can even displace organs and contribute to the formation of wrinkles. A better kind of aerobic exercise is found in passive, but high-energy, activities such as vigorous walking, swimming, bicycling, and skating. Gyms and spas offer workouts on treadmills, bike machines, Nordic-Tracks, stair climbers, ski machines, and even machines that duplicate swimming exercise without water! There are lots of ways to enjoy an active lifestyle that help you drop pounds.

Exercise is indeed the dieter's best friend, not just because it burns calories, but also because physiologically it is the fastest way to change metabolism, to cause a shift in the amount of food that is converted to energy and muscle rather than to fat. Moreover, exercise not only burns energy, but it keeps your metabolic rate high for up to four hours after you have finished. This means you are still expending energy long after you have finished your workout. To convert food and stored fat to energy, we need the oxygen derived from exercise. Without it, we feel tired and lazy because we cannot produce enough energy.

The kind and amount of exercise needed to knock off excess weight varies from person to person. A standard recommendation is to exercise five days a week at a level that will increase your heart rate for thirty minutes.

Now that you've found the Hippocrates Program, the nonsense is over. You can stop playing the diet yo-yo game, paying hundreds of dollars each year and risking your health on fad diets that allow you plenty of fattening and disease-promoting foods. What you need is nourishment and enzymes, not starvation. The Hippocrates Program will change the quality of what you eat by letting whole vegetables, fruits, sprouts, and greens replace fattening foods such as butter, cheese, eggs, red meats, and refined oils and sugar, as well as many high-fat vegetarian foods. And it will make exercise a natural part of your life and weight-loss program.

WEIGHT GAIN AND MAINTENANCE

Discussions of weight control tend to focus on weight loss and ignore the fact that there are thousands of people with lean body builds who don't want to lose weight and many more who are underweight or who have lost weight after an extended illness. The Hippocrates Health Program addresses these needs also. One should eat heavier living foods and develop muscle mass through resistance exercise.

Just Right

If you have a body size that you feel is just right for your age and height, the Hippocrates diet will supply you with the daily energy needed to maintain that weight. You may find, however, that you lose some weight during the first few weeks. This happens because the body is getting rid of waste weight: fat, calcium deposits, and toxins. Cleaning out the junk can cause a reduction in weight. But then, as the muscles begin to redevelop through healthy nutrition and resistance exercises, you'll see your body weight return to normal (with improved body shape!). During this period, you may want to follow the guidelines for gaining weight described below until your normal weight returns and stabilizes.

Building Up

After the initial period of detoxification that occurs when you first begin the Hippocrates diet (see chapter 6 for details about detoxification), the Hippocrates Program can help you gain weight—and build up your body strength and vitality at the same time. Too many underweight people feast on high-fat foods hoping to gain extra pounds, and thus good health. But they don't realize that the body can't regain vitality if no nutrients are in these foods and if the cell's ability to absorb nutrients is diminished by lack of enzymes and oxygen in the food.

Weight gain on the Hippocrates Program is based on a two-part plan: increased energy unit intake and resistance exercises. You'll want to make sure that your daily diet includes hefty portions of nutritious, high-energy foods such as avocados, sprouted grains and beans, seeds, and nuts. Select recipes in chapter 11 that include these ingredients. (Be sure to try sprouted grain breads and bean meals.) The foods' high-energy quotient and high nutrition will give your body what it needs to gain weight.

Weight Gain and Exercise

When weight gain is your goal, aerobic exercise is not your friend. You don't want to burn energy while you exercise—you want to build strong body muscle. That's why strength training (also called resistance training) should be part of your daily health program. Today, free weights (such as barbells) and/or resistance equipment (such as Nautilus or Universal equipment) are common in virtually all gyms and spas. Other forms of resistance exercises such as swimming against a current or with water weights and fins, isometrics, and Callanetics let you vary your routine for enjoyment and body growth.

You can also use your own body weight for resistance exercises. Push-ups, pull-ups, abdominal exercises, back extensions, and jumping rope are simple ways to effectively build body strength. These exercises build the muscles in the torso, legs, arms, and back by using gravity and functional movements. When doing resistance exercises briskly—with a count of four or five seconds in-between them—you also gain aerobic benefits without weight loss.

The benefits of resistance exercises are well worth the effort. They include the following:

- improved muscular strength and power
- a toned, rather than flabby, body appearance
- reduction and prevention of osteoporosis
- improved local muscular endurance
- improved strength and balance around the joints
- improved total body strength
- protection against injury
- a faster recovery time when injured

This list is not complete, of course, without mention of increased body weight. The firm, strengthened muscle weighs more than the weak flabby one. So without putting on more fat, you can increase your weight and improve your appearance.

Resistance exercises are best performed three times a week for thirty minutes each time. Begin using light weights with rapid movements; then slowly increase the weight.

THE PSYCHOLOGY OF FOOD

Thousands of weight-loss and weight-gain diets have failed because they did not take into account the mental and emotional connection we all have to food. It's too simple to say, "Just eat less and you'll lose weight." If it were that easy, there wouldn't be a billion-dollar industry built up around people's battle with food. Food symbolizes many things to different people—love, reward, solace, celebration, a family bond, and so on. All of these emotional factors influence how we deal with our body weight and image. In addition to its recommendations regarding diet and exercise, The Hippocrates Health Program adds this psychological component to its weight management plan.

For overeaters, the need to eat often comes not from a physical hunger but from an emotional hunger. It's our hearts that need the nourishment, our souls that need to be fed. We swallow our disappointments, we swallow our hurt, we swallow our anger, we swallow our pride. We eat when we're excited. We eat when we're sad, when we have too much to do or not enough to do. When our pain is intense, eating soothes us, or so we think. But it doesn't. It creates a pain all its own. It only prolongs the misery. But we blot this out, obsessed only with the very real, transitory pleasure it offers. Undereaters, on the other hand, "treat" their pain by dieting, yet only end up with a body that is weak and thin.

The Hippocrates Program doesn't ask you to change your personality or to stop eating. But it does give you the information you need to see food in a positive, life-sustaining and enhancing way. It reinforces that all-important premise that food is not the enemy— it is our ally in pursuit of health and longevity. On the Hippocrates Program, you will support your body in its effort to return to its healthy, vibrant shape by cleansing your body of toxins; by giving yourself permission to deal with your emotions (through relaxation techniques, psychological strengthening, and exercise); by using food for life-giving nourishment, not abusing it for emotional needs; and by feeding your body pure, unadulterated food that can be easily transformed into the nutrients you've been starving for. By living on living foods, you'll be able to abandon the debilitating body-image consciousness. Old eating habits will be broken. Emotions will no longer dictate what and how much you eat.

If weight management is one of your reasons for seeking a new diet and lifestyle, you can meet your goals by following the Hippocrates Program outlined in this book. Eat any of the foods recommended in chapters 6 and 8, make up a batch of the sprouts and green juices recommended in chapter 9, and enjoy any recipe in chapter 11. The same program that gives general wellness also offers superior weight management.

6

Becoming a
Living-Foods Vegetarian

Many people come to living-foods vegetarianism from a diet full of
meat, dairy, poultry, and fish, and almost all are hooked on cooked
and processed foods. Although these diets are not healthful, I realize that
people become psychologically attached to eating habits, and so it's not
easy to make a quick change to the Hippocrates diet. In most cases if
you are not in a life-threatening health crisis, and you're uncomfortable
about instantly changing your past eating habits, you can make a steady,
unhurried transfer to the Hippocrates Health Program.

A SIX-MONTH PLAN

Try mapping out a six-month plan. Your first steps must be to eliminate your addictions to caffeine, sugar, nicotine, alcohol and/or drugs.
Even many health-conscious vegetarians stumble on this tenet of
living-foods vegetarianism, but elimination of these poisons is
absolutely necessary.

Caffeine, sugar, nicotine, alcohol, and drugs are harmful pollutants that destroy nutrients and raise the impurity level of the blood. They also leave waste in the body that must be cleaned up by white blood cells. Rather than attend to their regular duty of maintaining good health, the white blood cells are overtaxed and their efficiency is weakened when they are diverted to cleaning out the debris left behind by these substances. These immunity robbers all must be eliminated from your diet. The one "bad" thing you hold on to is so often the biggest detriment to your health.

At the same time you're ditching bad habits, begin introducing living foods into your diet each day. Gradually increase the amount of your intake so that the percentage of living foods soon becomes greater than any other foods. Then, if you haven't already, start eliminating meat and dairy products by reducing the number of weekly meals that rely on these products. Plan your shopping and menus in advance (see chapters 8 and 11), so you're not stuck with "nothing" to eat and tempted to grab the nearest piece of dead food. On this plan, you will not see rapid progress, but will notice gradual, definitive, and long-lasting differences in how you feel.

PERSONALIZING THE PROGRAM

Your body will tell you how strictly you should adhere to a living-foods diet to achieve physical wellness. To reverse serious health problems almost always requires an initial 100 percent adherence to the Hippocrates diet of living, organic fruits, vegetables, grains, sprouts, beans, nuts, and seeds. However, if you are fairly healthy and want to pursue productive longevity, it may be harmless to indulge in a carefully selected variety of cooked foods (like whole grain pastas, beans, grains, and steamed vegetables). Through long-term studies of enzyme and oxygen levels, we have discovered that a healthy body has the ability to maintain health if no more than one-quarter of the food eaten each day is cooked. If you can consistently make living foods at least 75 percent (by weight) of your daily intake, your

Figure 6-1 This is an example of an easy meal that follows the living foods lifestyle.

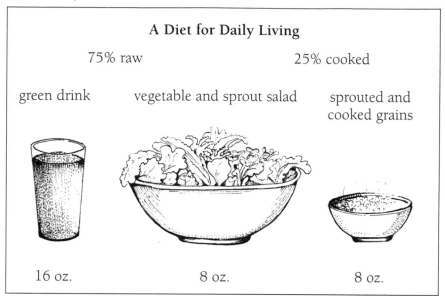

A Diet for Daily Living

75% raw   25% cooked

green drink   vegetable and sprout salad   sprouted and
                                                          cooked grains

16 oz.   8 oz.   8 oz.

dedication to achieving total body health will bring rewards that know no bounds.

WHAT CAN I EAT?

A diet of living foods is not a Spartan diet, but it does require a change from the more common, processed Western diet you may be used to. Again, like vegan-vegetarians, living-food vegetarians elimi-nate all animal and dairy products; then they go two steps further by 1) eliminating junk and processed foods, and 2) by eating at least 75 percent of their foods uncooked.

This diet contains all the foods of nature that the human body was meant to thrive on (including green drinks, which are made of foods like cucumber, parsley, celery, watercress, and sprouts). A partial list includes the following.

Fresh Vegetables

The majority percentage of your daily diet should come from fresh vegetables like these:

Salad Greens

arugula
bok choy
chicory
collard greens
dandelion
garlic greens
kale
lettuces
mustard greens
scallions
spinach
Swiss chard
turnip greens
watercress
sunflower
    greens

Sprouts and Baby Greens

adzuki
alfalfa
buckwheat lettuce
clover
fenugreek
chickpeas
garlic
lentil
mung bean sprouts
mustard
onion
pea greens
radish
sprouted bean mix

Roots and Tubers

beets
burdock root
carrots
daikon radish
garlic
ginger
leeks
onion
parsnips
red radish
rutabaga
sweet potatoes
turnips
yams

Vegetables

asparagus
bell peppers
broccoli
cabbage
cauliflower
celery
corn
cucumbers
green beans
mushrooms
peas (fresh)
summer squashes
winter squashes
zucchini

Fresh Herbs

basil
chives
cilantro
dill
mint
oregano
parsley
sage
savory
sorrel
tarragon
thyme

Sea Vegetables

alaria
arame
dulse
hijiki
kelp
nori
wakame

Fruits

No more than 15 percent of your diet should come from fruit. Even organic fruits are often picked unripe and contain too much sugar.

Best	Okay Occasionally	Best Not Eaten*
apples	avocado	apricots
bananas	berries	coconut, brown
cherries (deep red)	cantaloupe	dates
grapes	cherimoya	dried fruit
kiwi	grapefruit	mangoes
lemons	honeydew melon	oranges
papaya	persimmons (soft)	peaches
pears	pineapple	plums
watermelon	sapote	
	starfruit	
	tangerine	

*These fruits too often are harvested before they are ripened and so lack the essential vitamins and minerals that would have been manufactured in the tree-ripening process. Also, dates and dried fruits are too sweet.

Seeds, Legumes, Whole Grains, and Nuts

Ten percent (by weight) of the daily diet should be from seeds, legumes, whole grains, and nuts. All items in these lists should be purchased raw and then germinated and/or sprouted before eating or cooking.

Seeds	Legumes	Nuts
flaxseed	adzuki beans	almonds
pumpkin	chickpeas	coconut, green
sesame	lentils	filberts
sunflower	lima beans	pecans
	mung beans	walnuts
	peas, green or yellow	
	pinto beans	
	Northern white beans	

Whole Grains*

amaranth (3)
basmati rice (-)
buckwheat (hulled) (5)
millet (1)
quinoa (2)
rye (-)
spelt (-)
teff (4)

*Numbers following grains are in the order of preferred usage (1 being most preferred). Those with no numbers should be used sparingly.

These abundant raw foods make up the recommended 75 percent living foods of the Hippocrates Program: 60 percent sprouts and vegetables, 15 percent fruits, and 10 percent seeds, nuts, grains, and legumes. The remaining 15 percent will come from a variety of foods easily found in health food stores. In chapter 8, you'll find a long list of these items that will fill your cravings for "foods" such as potato chips, pizza, hot dogs, cheese, milk, bagels, peanut butter, soft drinks, chocolate, and sugar. You'll come to see that the Hippocrates diet isn't a trial by sacrifice, but rather a challenge of change. It's time to look in new directions for the foods your body needs.

FEELING CHANGE BEFORE YOU FEEL BETTER

During the first week of the program at Hippocrates, I often hear people say, "I'm eating all this healthy food and I feel lousy. I don't understand it." What they don't understand is how the body rids itself of the toxic waste left behind by animal products and cooked and processed foods filled with chemical pollutants. When you first begin a living-foods diet, these wastes are discharged from the cells, organs, arteries, and veins into the bloodstream for removal from the body. But before they leave, they may make one last cry that you may hear as symptoms of illness.

This internal cleansing is a lot like house cleaning. Have you ever walked into a house that had been tightly closed up and left untouched for a few years? Things often look relatively clean and in order—until you take out the broom and suddenly stir up a dust storm. If you then get out a pail of water and a scrub brush and create scattered puddles of muddy water, you might well find yourself sitting in the middle of the room, wondering if your efforts are worth the mess you've created.

So it goes with the body. There's no doubt it's worth the effort, but you may experience symptoms that can be discouraging unless you understand what is actually going on. The toxins being discarded are saving you from more serious disease that would result if you keep them in your body too much longer—possibly hepatitis, kidney disorders, blood disease, heart disease, arthritis, nerve degenerations, or even cancer.

While the body is busy using the enzymes and oxygen of living foods to clean up the mess from deep within each and every cell, these are some of the uncomfortable reactions that are possible:

increased flatulence	aches and pains
skin eruptions	fever
increased thirst	weakness
cravings	diarrhea
runny nose	edema
headaches	nausea
irritability	cold and flu symptoms
constipation	bad breath
insomnia	dizziness
nervousness	frequent urination
coated tongue	nightmares
fatigue	loss of appetite

The symptoms will vary according to the toxins being discarded and the condition of the organs involved in the elimination. If you have eaten healthy cooked foods and have avoided body-abusers such as caffeine, nicotine, sugar, and alcohol in the past, your detox-ification symptoms may be quite mild. If you are making a drastic switch in diet and lifestyle, your symptoms may be quite severe.

The good news is that detoxification is a sign that your body is becoming younger and healthier every day because you are throwing off more and more wastes that would eventually have brought pain, disease, and suffering. The majority of people find their reactions tol-erable and are able to bear with them motivated by the promise of vitality, health, and longevity.

The length of the cleansing process depends on how many years you have abused your body with a poor diet. The noticeable detox-ification period usually lasts for only a week or two, with little to great intensity. It will continue for years with characteristic, but far less noticeable, ups and downs until you reach the seven-year point when the body has fully regenerated. (See "The Three Phases of the Hippocrates Health Program" on page 119 for details about the seven-year cycles.) But certainly, even right from the start, you will notice a reduction in the intensity of your detox symptoms as your body becomes accustomed to your new living-foods diet.

Major Organs of Elimination

Although every cell of the body has "workers" that assist in removing waste from the cell, certain organs specialize in waste management. Below are these major organs and ways that you can assist them during the initial detoxification period.

Colon.   The colon is the solid-waste management organ in the body. Medical specialists have found individuals who have up to eighty pounds of mucous and rubberlike waste impacted along the wall of this organ. Cleaning out the colon can be a tough job.

You can support your colon's efforts to rid itself of stored waste with colon hydrotherapies that use wheatgrass juice implants (see page 134). These are highly effective in reducing negative cleansing reactions.

Kidneys.   The kidneys are the water management organs. The kidneys are responsible for keeping the chemistry of the blood alkaline by filtering out the dissolved acid wastes.

You can assist your kidneys by drinking plenty of purified water and fresh alkaline juices. Consume a minimum of one-half ounce alkaline juice per pound of body weight on a daily basis. Alkaline juices include cucumber juice, celery juice, sunflower green juice, and buckwheat sprout green juice.

Liver.   The liver is the recycling center of the body. This organ sorts out toxins and sends them to the appropriate organ for elimination. If the principle elimination organ is backed up, the liver will redirect the toxins as best it can.

Wheatgrass implants (see page 134) offer a direct shot in the arm to the liver and help it pull toxins out of the blood more quickly.

Lungs.   The lungs are the blood's air purifier. They introduce oxygen directly into the bloodstream and, at the same time, remove waste gases that are produced in every cell of the body.

Deep breathing from the diaphragm is most helpful to the lungs. It's also important to breathe in smog-free oxygen. If you live in the city, try to find an oxygen-rich environment where you can perform aerobic exercises.

Lymph.   The lymph glands are the major "garbage arteries" in the body. This intricate network of tubing is the one that carries the bulk of waste from the cells of the body to the final elimination organs. Major lymphatic glands are the appendix, spleen, thymus, and tonsils. These glands tend to swell during detoxification.

Regular exercise (both aerobic and resistance) and massage are beneficial to the lymphatic system. Drink plenty of fluids to help dilute and transport the toxins through the body.

Skin.   The skin is the elimination organ with the largest surface area. In addition to regulating temperature and body moisture content, the skin often functions as a backup for the other elimination organs. If the colon is clogged, for example, toxins may try to escape through skin rashes, acne, and other skin disorders.

Exercise, dry skin brushing (see page 138), massage, and drinking plenty of fluids all encourage the skin to breathe, perspire and thus release toxins.

General Detoxification Tonics

If you begin to feel symptoms of detoxification, try the following antidotes:

1. Upon waking, drink lemon water (mix the juice of one lemon in eight ounces of water) with up to one-half teaspoon of cayenne pepper. This helps to open up the circulatory system and alkalinize the body fluids, increasing the rate of detoxification.
2. Fast one day every week, consuming only freshly-squeezed green drinks (see page 177), vegetable juices, purified water, and herbal teas. These fasting days will allow any potential long-term toxins to be released before they can cause serious damage. It's like changing your oil *before* your engine fails due to wear-and-tear.
3. Exercise daily. Aerobic, resistance, and stretching exercises speed the elimination process.
4. Do not treat your detoxification symptoms with drugs or vitamins. Detoxification symptoms are part of a healing process. Don't try to heal a symptom of healing.
5. Let fevers below 103 degrees run their course. A fever is an indication that the body is working overtime to cleanse the body.
6. Rest. The body needs energy to dispel toxins. The more you rest and sleep when the symptoms are present, the milder they are and the more quickly they are terminated.

Becoming sick is the body's only way to eliminate a buildup of excess toxins. When you feel the effects of this detoxification, don't worry—cheer your body's efforts knowing you will come through with greater vitality, energy, and overall good health.

THE THREE PHASES OF THE HIPPOCRATES HEALTH PROGRAM

The Hippocrates Health Program is divided into three, seven-year phases. When you become a living-foods vegetarian, you take the first step into this twenty-one-year expedition that ultimately will bring you to the peak of physical/mental, emotional, and spiritual health.

Mind/body health is the foundation upon which you will thrive for the rest of your life, and it is the focus of this book. But there's more; take a moment to look at where the Hippocrates Health Program can take you.

Phase 1: What Am I Made Of?

In Phase 1, you rebuild and revitalize your physical being by nurturing the cells of your body with electrically charged, living foods and exercise. You come to understand the answer to the question, "What am I made of?" Although complete physical wellness takes a full seven years to attain, within a few weeks you'll see physical changes that clearly show improvement in your health . You'll notice:

- a stronger physique
- a more flexible body
- greater mobility and agility
- improved functioning of the digestive system
- weight regulation
- reduced cholesterol levels
- greater awareness, perception, and sensitivity

These physical changes are the result of certain biochemical reactions within and among the trillions of cells in the body. The regeneration of these cells, the restructuring of bone, reestablishment of proper circulation, and the renewal of every bodily function virtually changes the physical makeup of the body. That's why even terminal diseases can be turned around.

But complete renewal takes time. Although the cells are constantly regenerating (giving us completely new lungs in seventy days and a new heart in thirty days, for example), the cell mutation and degeneration that bring on disease and ill health have their own rhythm and won't totally disappear from the cell structure when it renews itself. But on a living-foods diet, the mutant, weak, and/or oxygen-starved cells slowly return to normal as each regenerative cycle passes, over the course of seven years. While the affected cells themselves are renewing, the disorder can not spread or exacerbate further because the tissues around them are no longer weak or vulnerable; they have become strong and resistant. So the cancer, or the fibroid, or the calcium deposit, or the virus, can't progress or maintain its hold in the body.

Phase 2: Who Am I?

After seven years on a living-foods diet, the body is physically rejuvenated. At this time, you'll be ready to enter into the second seven-year phase of wellness that brings emotional health. Emotional health must wait for this second phase to be completed because the potential for true emotional stability is possible only when the physical needs of the body have been met. Physical health gives us the strength and openness to look deeper into our hearts and souls to answer the question, "Who am I?"

During the second seven years on the Hippocrates Health Program, you can expect to attain the following:

• the desire to be actively involved in life, rather than watch from the sidelines
• the ability to focus

- the drive to create and reach goals
- improved relationships
- a larger view and vision of the future

Phase 3: Why Am I Here?

The third part of the Hippocrates Program brings you to the spiritual phase. Once you have the answers to the questions "What am I made of?" (the first physical phase), and "Who am I?" (the second emotional phase), you're ready to venture an answer to the question, "Why am I here?" (the spiritual phase). Spiritual life is more than any religious training we might have experienced; it empowers who we are every second of our lives, what we're going to do, and where we're going. In this third cycle of the program, we have a greater ability to move forward with our spiritual life because we've met our physical and emotional needs.

In Retrospect

I can see these seven-year cycles very clearly in my own life. Having been a living-foods vegetarian for well over twenty-one years, I can look back and see how the evolutionary process unfolded. The only sadness I see in retrospect is that this cycle is a normal process that should have started at birth. In the first seven years of life, we should build our physical base; in the second seven years, we should nurture emotional growth in the quest to understand who we are; by the time we reach the age of 21, we should be ready to answer the question, "Why am I here?" But because we are distracted in youth by processed, cooked, and junk foods that keep us from building the first base of physical health, we have to start this journey as an adult. But once on the road, we should never look back. We should look forward to the time when we will have finally attained the promise of physical, emotional, and spiritual health.

As you change your eating habits to meet your body's needs, you automatically begin to build the physical base you'll need to pursue emotional and spiritual growth. Becoming a living-foods vegetarian brings you not only personal health but also begins an awakening process that will show you the interrelatedness of all humans and the world we live in.

7

Getting the Most from the Hippocrates Health Program

Anyone who eats a diet of living foods automatically improves his or her health, slows aging, gains mental clarity, and boosts immune power. But the Hippocrates Health Program includes more than just diet. Other aspects of the program when combined with a living-foods diet guarantee absolute, optimal results. In addition to changing your diet, we recommend the following be done: careful food combining; fasting; colon cleansing; exercise; dry skin brushing; aromatherapy; taking saunas, steam baths, and whirlpools; massage; and electrical frequency and laser therapy.

FOOD COMBINING

One goal of the Hippocrates diet is to bring foods into the body that allow quick absorption of nutrients and quick elimination of waste. At the institute, I give a lecture that explains to our guests how the combination of foods eaten at one sitting can either hinder or help this process. Even if you eat a meal that is 100 percent living foods, you will lose some of the healthy benefits if those foods do not combine well in the digestive tract.

The principles of food combining are these:

1. Foods are made up of natural chemicals. Our bodies are similar to test tubes in a laboratory. As in chemistry experiments, if the right elements are combined, reactions ranging from sedative to explosive can be created. Starchy foods, for example, require alkaline digestive juices, initially supplied in the mouth. Protein foods require the acidic juices formed in the stomach. When the acids mix with the alkaline juices they tend to neutralize each other. Thus, the mixing of starches and protein foods at the same meal slows digestion of both, and indigestion occurs.

2. Foods digest at a different rate in different acid/alkaline environments. This can be compared to automobiles that have different acceleration and top-end speeds. If you put a slow vehicle in front of a faster one on a one-lane road, the faster one will have to slow down in order to prevent an accident. When you do this with food in the digestive system, the "faster" food runs into the "slow" food and causes a crash in the form of indigestion, bloating, and poor assimilation.

The Basic Food Combining Groups

The following pages show lists of foods grouped together according to speed of digestion (from fastest to slowest). Foods with similar digestion times should be eaten together, while foods with different times should be eaten at separate meals. These are only a sampling of foods. You can eat many more foods; just try to categorize them by type as indicated.

15 to 30 Minutes: Wheatgrass

Wheatgrass (fully discussed in chapter 9) should be taken on an empty stomach or before meals. It can be used alone or with other vegetable and fruit juices.

15 to 30 Minutes: Melons

Melons should always be eaten alone because they digest quickly. When combined with other fruits (say, in a fruit salad), their digestion is delayed by the slowly digested fruits, and this can cause fermentation. Melons include cantaloupe, crenshaw, honeydew, watermelon, etc.

1 to 4 Hours: Fruits

Although some fruits besides melons have approximately the same digestion speed, they should not all be eaten together. Acid, subacid, and sweet fruits each have a different water and sugar content and are more easily digested when eaten with fruits of similar type.

Acid fruits (1–1½ hours):   grapefruits, lemons, oranges, pomegranates, pineapples, strawberries

Subacid fruits (1½–2 hours):   apples, apricots, most berries, grapes, kiwi, mangoes, pears, peaches, sweet cherries

Sweet fruits (4 hours):   bananas, all dried fruit, persimmons

2 to 3 Hours: Vegetables

Sprouted greens: alfalfa, arugula, buckwheat, cabbage, clover, garlic, kale, lentil, mung bean, mustard, radish, sunflower

Fruit vegetables: cucumbers, red bell peppers, summer squash, zucchini

Leafy greens: arugula, bok choy, cabbage, chard, collards, kale, lettuce, mizuna, mustard greens, scallions, spinach, watercress

Low-starch root vegetables: beets, burdock, carrots, parsnips, radishes, turnips

3 Hours: Starches

Sprouted grains: amaranth, barley, millet, quinoa, rye, teff, wheat

Sprouted legumes: chickpeas, lentils, peas

Winter squashes: acorn, butternut, hubbard, kabocha, spaghetti

Potatoes: sweet potatoes, yams

4 Hours: Protein

Seeds: pumpkin, sesame, sunflower

Nuts: almonds, Brazil nuts, hazel, pecans, pine nuts, walnuts (no peanuts or cashews; they contain a low-grade oil that is extremely difficult to digest)

The best way to combine food is to choose foods from the same group at each meal. If you do mix groups, remember these guidelines suggested by the Hippocrates Institute:

- Fruits and vegetables do not mix. The sugars and acids in fruits slow the digestion of the carbohydrates in vegetables and can cause fermentation, bloating, and gas. It is best to eat fruits and vegetables separately at different meals. Occasional fruit desserts can be eaten 2 hours after a meal of vegetables or sprouts.
- When eating fruits, avoid mixing acid fruits with sweet fruits. If you must mix fruits, combine either sweet or acid fruits with subacid fruits. Limit fruit to no more than 15 percent of your diet.
- All greens, sprouts, and vegetables (including avocados) mix well together. Sauces made from avocados, seeds, or nuts also mix well with greens, vegetables, and sprouts. But to avoid using overly complex mixtures of these foods at one meal. A good rule of thumb is to limit the number of foods used in combination to five or fewer.

- Avoid eating breads, sprouted grains, or grain crisps with fruits.
- Try to avoid drinking with your meals. It is better to take juices 15 to 30 minutes before meals or 2 to 3 hours after. Drinking while eating weakens the action of the digestive juices; it is also unnecessary to slake thirst when you eat plenty of natural foods because they have a high water content.
- At each meal, eat raw food before any cooked food. Otherwise the cooked food holds up the digestion of the raw, causing it to ferment and produce uncomfortable gas.

Good Combinations

- protein and sprouts and leafy greens
- starch and sprouts and vegetables
- fruit from one category

Poor Combinations

- fruit and starch
- fruit and protein
- fruit and vegetables
- starch and protein

(Avocados, onion, and garlic are the only exception to the fruit/vegetable rule. They are easily combined with either fruits or vegetables, making them a truly versatile and important food.)

The art of proper food combining takes time to master because it challenges some of our established notions about "good" foods. Take an all-natural granola bar, for example: granola usually contains rolled oats (starch), nuts (protein), and honey (sugar) and dried fruit (sweet fruit) in a disastrously tasty combination. The protein mixed with starch creates various gasses, including sulfur. The combination of starch and sweet fruit creates fermentation and alcohol.

With practice and patience, soon you'll be selecting your foods not only for their nutritional value but for their benefits in combination.

Figure 7-1 Food combining.

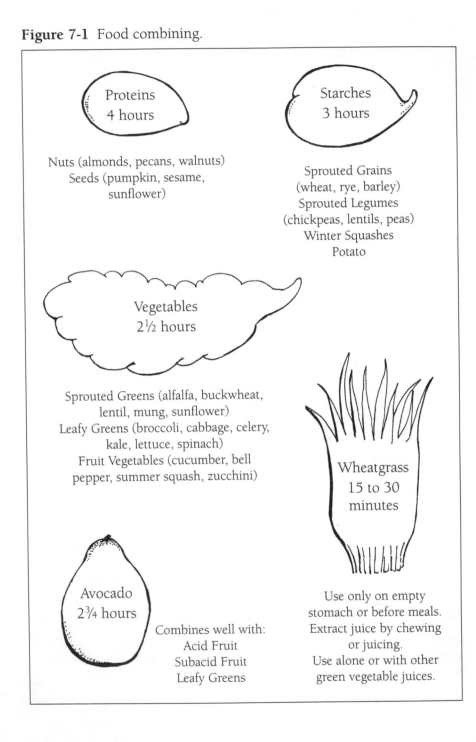

Proteins
4 hours

Nuts (almonds, pecans, walnuts)
Seeds (pumpkin, sesame,
sunflower)

Starches
3 hours

Sprouted Grains
(wheat, rye, barley)
Sprouted Legumes
(chickpeas, lentils, peas)
Winter Squashes
Potato

Vegetables
2½ hours

Sprouted Greens (alfalfa, buckwheat,
lentil, mung, sunflower)
Leafy Greens (broccoli, cabbage, celery,
kale, lettuce, spinach)
Fruit Vegetables (cucumber, bell
pepper, summer squash, zucchini)

Wheatgrass
15 to 30
minutes

Avocado
2¾ hours

Combines well with:
Acid Fruit
Subacid Fruit
Leafy Greens

Use only on empty
stomach or before meals.
Extract juice by chewing
or juicing.
Use alone or with other
green vegetable juices.

Figure 7-1 Food combining (*continued*).

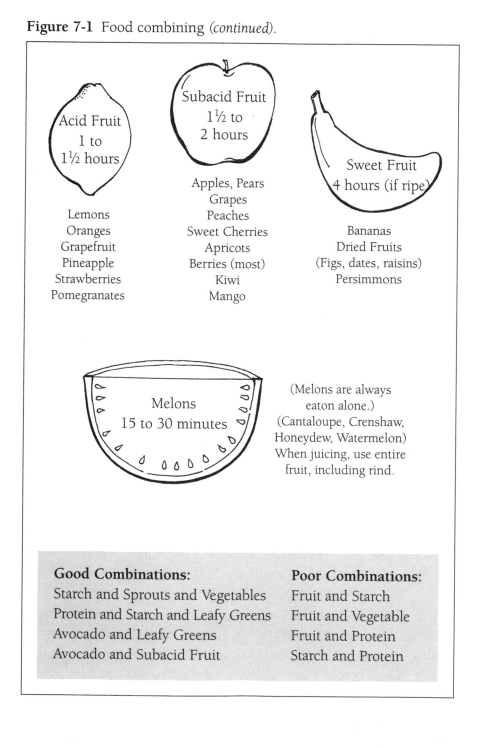

Acid Fruit
1 to
1½ hours

Lemons
Oranges
Grapefruit
Pineapple
Strawberries
Pomegranates

Subacid Fruit
1½ to
2 hours

Apples, Pears
Grapes
Peaches
Sweet Cherries
Apricots
Berries (most)
Kiwi
Mango

Sweet Fruit
4 hours (if ripe)

Bananas
Dried Fruits
(Figs, dates, raisins)
Persimmons

Melons
15 to 30 minutes

(Melons are always
eaton alone.)
(Cantaloupe, Crenshaw,
Honeydew, Watermelon)
When juicing, use entire
fruit, including rind.

Good Combinations:
Starch and Sprouts and Vegetables
Protein and Starch and Leafy Greens
Avocado and Leafy Greens
Avocado and Subacid Fruit

Poor Combinations:
Fruit and Starch
Fruit and Vegetable
Fruit and Protein
Starch and Protein

FASTING

I believe that most disease begins with an accumulation of toxins and negative emotional/mental blockages. As a result, energy can be deeply locked within the body. But by following the Hippocrates Program and fasting one day every week, you can unlock the physical energy and allow it to penetrate and strengthen the emotional, mental, and spiritual areas. Throughout history, many great leaders, both spiritual and political, have used fasting as a mechanism to accelerate their health and understanding.

While most natural health proponents accept the benefits of fasting, two distinct schools of thought debate the process, with some convincing arguments on each side. One group strongly supports water fasting, arguing that taking any other type of liquid nourishment cannot be considered authentic. On the other hand, I believe that fasting with vegetable and sprout juices brings far better results, without the severe reactions that often accompany water fasts. Drinking only water greatly accelerates the cleansing process, causing massive amounts of toxins to be released from the body. This puts unnecessary stress on the organs of elimination. Juice fasting, while just as effective, causes less trauma and discomfort. And more important, on a juice fast you are nourished and strengthened instead of being depleted and weakened.

Getting Started

The first questions our guests usually ask about fasting are these:

1. What do I drink on my day of fasting?
Our experience and research indicates that for optimum results, green drinks (see recipes in chapter 11) should be the principal drink during the day. These drinks can be supplemented with purified lemon

water, watermelon or cucumber juice, herbal teas, or small amounts of diluted freshly-squeezed fruit juice.

2. How much should I drink during the day?
I suggest consuming at least two quarts (eight 8-ounce glasses) during the day. Most of this should be consumed during the morning hours with the last drink taken at least three hours before retiring for the night, if possible.

3. When and what should I eat on the day following the fast?
Upon waking, consume liquid. If you do not have a sensitivity to sugar, try watermelon, apple, or pear juice mixed ⅓ juice to ⅔ water. If you are sugar-sensitive, try cucumber or squash juice or light herbal teas such as chamomile or spearmint. This allows your body to finish its housecleaning tasks. The first meal should be light. The best choices are a piece of tree-ripened fruit or some sprouts and light vegetables; these give your digestive system a chance to wake up gently. You may eat as soon as thirty minutes after your morning drink. For lunch and dinner, you may resume your customary eating program.

When It's Over

When the fast is over, you may want to know more about fasting. Common questions include these:

1. I was tired, achy, and irritable most of the day. Is this normal?
During the first few one-day fasts, this reaction can be expected. This is simply the release and elimination of stored toxins from the cells. Celebrate these experiences that signal the expulsion of disease-causing poisons. You can minimize these experiences by increasing the amount of liquid you consume during the day, especially the green drinks.

2. How often should I repeat this one-day fast?
Once every week. Choose a day when you have minimal demands on you and allow your body, mind, and spirit to take you where it wants to as you clean out. It will also enhance your performance on the other six days of the week. People who follow this program report that their fasting day becomes the most productive of the week. If you are ill and debilitated or have a blood sugar problem, use a clean mono-diet on your fasting day—for example, only green salad and extra juice.

3. Can I extend the fast beyond one day?
Only consider doing this if you are in good health—and then only up to three days maximum. If you feel you want to extend a fast beyond three days, you should locate a reputable fasting resort staffed with a professional to guide you well.

Fasting Menu

You should think of your fast day as being like any other day except that you are juicing your living food rather than eating it. A sample menu for a fasting day might be like the following:

Breakfast:
watermelon or cucumber juice (seeds and rind included) or juice of apples, grapes, pears, and berries. (Except for watermelon juice, dilute fruit juices one part juice with two parts water.)

In-Between:
purified water, lemon water, or herb tea as often as desired

Lunch:
Green drink/vegetable juices

In-Between:
water, lemon water, or herb tea as often as needed

Dinner:
green drink/ vegetable juices
(Try not to drink again after dinner.)

Give It a Try

Fasting is not required on the Hippocrates Health Plan, but it complements your efforts to obtain optimal health. Give yourself the opportunity to experience the liberation and lightness that liquid nourishment days will bring you. Thomas Edison, Albert Einstein, Mohandas Gandhi, Franklin D. Roosevelt and many others used this simple process for purification and enlightenment.

COLON CLEANSING

There's no debate at all in medical literature: You need a clean and healthy colon to assimilate nutrients and dispose of waste. Yet millions of people have colons that are congested, twisted out of shape, and impacted with toxic waste. This can cause a multitude of bowel disorders and chronic diseases. This isn't surprising—even though a person may have a bowel movement daily, there may still be several days' or even a week's worth of waste inside the colon. A badly impacted colon can be carrying an excess of ten pounds of fecal matter at one time. This provides a breeding ground for unfriendly bacteria that can cause problems such as headaches, flatulence, indigestion, colitis, and bowel cancer. When these wastes accumulate, the colon becomes weak and sluggish, causing constipation. The accumulations tend to harden in the pockets of the colon walls. This hardened material obstructs the peristalsis (the natural muscular contractions of the bowel) and more and more buildup occurs. This, in turn, interferes with final absorption and digestion; instead of absorbing nutrients, the undigested food putrefies, creating toxic conditions.

Quick Tips for a Healthy Colon

To achieve a healthy colon, start with these three simple steps:

1. Respond to nature's call to eliminate. Try to establish a routine bowel movement first thing in the morning. All night, bowel functions have been active on the bacterial level and inactive on the metabolism level—they need relief in the morning. Repeat once more if possible.
2. Place a footstool or box under both feet when seated on the toilet. By raising the feet off the ground, you put yourself in a squatting position that is more natural and encourages easy elimination. (The design of the modern toilet has contributed to countless cases of constipation.)
3. Exercise. Exercise prevents the abdominal muscles from sagging and becoming weak. It brings oxygen-rich blood to the intestines, which gives the cells health and vitality. Exercise also stimulates peristalsis (but do not exercise immediately after eating because the process of digestion requires a great deal of energy).

Enemas and Implants

In addition to the three simple steps, enemas and implants help the colon regain normal muscle tone and strength. Enemas and implants are especially helpful during the first few weeks of your change in diet when waste matter is sent to the colon from all parts of the body for elimination.

The Enema. A full enema can be self-administered using a sterilized long colon tube attached to an enema bag filled with water (usually one to two quarts). While lying on your back with a pillow under your buttocks, insert the lubricated tube (do not force it farther than it will easily go). Allow the water to enter the colon slowly. Let in as much water as you can comfortably retain and dispel the water when you feel the urge (never force it to stay in).

The Implant.   Implants work to purge the colon and liver. They nourish the body via absorption in the colon; this keeps the electrolytes in the body healthy and strong. Follow an enema with an implant. To self-administer, fill the enema bag with at least four ounces of a fresh, high-chlorophyll liquid. This liquid may be wheat or barley grass juice. Blue-green algae and acidophilus powder dissolved in water, or green sprout juice (see chapter 11 for recipes) are not as powerful but at times may be used. Implant this juice in your colon using the enema procedure described above. Then remove the tube and remain lying down. Retain the implant for fifteen to twenty minutes before expelling it. Through years of research with guests at the Hippocrates Institute, I have found that enemas with implants actually restore a better electrolyte balance in the colon.

Colon Hydrotherapy

Some of our guests have bowels so badly impacted and damaged that they begin colon cleansing with colon hydrotherapy (colonics). A colonic is a continuous enema administered by a professional health-care provider. As water is continuously introduced into the full length of the colon, more and more pieces of hardened, putrefied waste are washed out. In most parts of the world, you can arrange to have a professional colonic treatment. Look for locations in health magazines or in your phone book.

EXERCISE

Many people equate exercise with only weight control, body contouring, flexibility, and muscular strength. Actually, cosmetic results are less important than the internal benefits.

The vascular, lymphatic, circulatory, digestive, immune, and respiratory systems are profoundly dependent upon physical activity for efficient functioning. And we benefit immensely on an emotional level, too, because exercise reduces stress, anxiety, lethargy, and depression.

An exercise program is part of the Hippocrates Health Plan. Vigorous exercise directly influences these three important functions of your bloodstream:

1. The bloodstream carries nutrients, extracted from the food you eat, to every cell in your body. Exercise helps speed these nutrients to their destination and at the same time brings enormous amounts of oxygen into the bloodstream. The highly oxygenated blood helps the nutrients or fuel to be burned more completely when it reaches the cell. In this way, exercise actually helps feed our cells.
2. The bloodstream is also the sanitation department, carrying off residues left over after the food/fuel has been burned. Every microscopic cell can be compared to a tiny engine where low-level combustion takes place, and this is why our bodies are warm. Although this explanation is admittedly simplistic, it does convey the idea that exercise keeps the blood flowing quickly, allowing residues and toxic wastes to be eliminated.
3. A fast-moving bloodstream keeps the veins and arteries open because it does not allow a buildup of cholesterol on their inside walls (when arteries and veins are clear of obstructions, blood pressure is normal).

An Exercise Program

An effective exercise program should place emphasis on overall body conditioning and should develop the major muscle groups of the body. If an area is ignored or overemphasized, this results in imbalance.

You should incorporate three kinds of exercise into your program:

Aerobic Training. By increasing your heart rate, aerobic training increases oxygen levels in every cell of the body, provides for more complete utilization of available nutrients, neutralizes toxins throughout the body, and improves the body's elimination processes. Outdoors, try bicycling, swimming, or walking. Indoors, try stair-climbing, treadmill, trampoline, or bicycling equipment.

Figure 7-2 Three types of exercise.

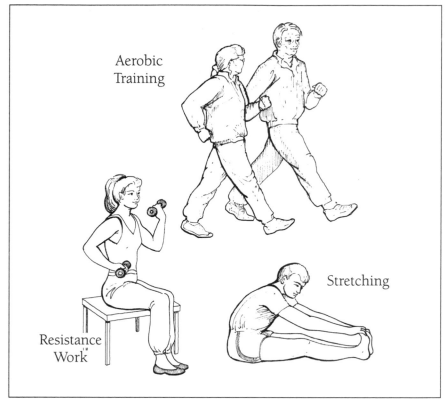

Stretching.   Stretching enables your joints and muscles to limber up and become more flexible. To stretch, slowly ease into the desired position (avoiding pain). Back off slightly from this stretch position and hold for ten to thirty seconds. Never bounce!

Resistance Work. Free weights and machines are the two most common tools for resistance exercise. Water resistance, noncompetitive gymnastics, and hatha yoga are some other examples. A combination of free weights, machines, and isometrics provide maximum results and variety. Heavy weights with few repetitions increase muscle mass. Lighter weights with more repetitions tone, rather than build, muscle mass.

Generally, muscles should be fatigued to gain the desired results. However, you should never demand so much from yourself during a workout that you feel excessive soreness the next day.

Schedule resistance or strength-training workouts three to four times each week (every other day is perfect). Daily workouts are not recommended except in the case of high-repetition, low-resistance work (such as exercises with ankle and wrist weights). On off-days, you can do low-impact aerobic exercises such as speed walking, swimming, the Stairmaster, or NordicTrack.

You can accomplish a great deal in thirty minutes, if the workout is at a sufficient level of intensity and if periods of rest between exercises are minimal.

Be sure you warm up before exercising. A warm-up should consist of three to five minutes of brisk walking, rope jumping, stationary cycling, or mild calisthenics to increase respiration, elevate body temperature, and stretch ligaments and connective tissue.

DRY SKIN BRUSHING

Your skin constantly breathes and eliminates toxins. (The average person eliminates about two pounds of waste through the skin each day!) If skin pores are blocked and can't function fully, the kidneys, liver, and lymphatic system will have to compensate and will be overloaded with toxins. A dry skin brushing just before showering—or in a steam bath or sauna—helps remove toxins from the pores and stimulates the lymphatic and circulatory system. Try it every day.

You'll need a long-handled, natural, hard bristle brush for the body and a soft one for the face and sensitive areas. Using both circular motions and straight strokes toward the heart, vigorously rub your entire skin surface beginning with your feet, including the soles, then moving up your legs, front and back, with firm sweeping strokes. Brush from your hands up your arms and across your shoulders, then brush your back and buttocks. On your front (abdomen, chest and neck) brush a little more gently. Not only does dry skin brushing help to clean out the average two pounds of waste that leave through the skin each day, it also rejuvenates.

AROMATHERAPY

Aromatherapy is a complementary therapy that strives for physical, mental, and spiritual health through the use of essential oils. Essential oils are natural aromatic liquid substances often considered to be the life forces of plants. These essences are capable of inducing a state of harmony and well-being in body, mind, and spirit and they can promote and maintain health by raising levels of resistance and immunity to disease.

Essential oils enter the body in one of two ways. They can be placed in misting units that dispense the fragrance throughout the room; the oil droplets are then inhaled and absorbed through the skin. The oils can also be rubbed directly onto the skin at selected pressure points. Whether in mist or liquid form, essential oils are able to penetrate through the skin due to their small molecules. They are then absorbed into the bloodstream and into the lymphatic system. They encourage the growth of new cells, thus delaying the process of aging by eliminating old cells more quickly. Here they stimulate various hormones to affect changes in the cells. Different oils affect different hormones, but the subtle changes that occur are the same: the weaker cells abandon the body and the remaining cells are stregthened. This delays the process of aging by encouraging the growth of new cells and eliminating old cells. Circulation can also be improved, pain relieved, fluid retention reduced, and nerves calmed and soothed.

Natural organic aromatic essences are extremely safe when used properly. They have an advantage over drugs because they are excreted, leaving no toxic residues behind. Side effects are virtually nonexistent. But because there are hundreds of essential oils—each with various health-promoting qualities—as well as oils that can be toxic if used incorrectly, it's wise to use aromatherapy under the supervision of someone trained in their use like a professional skin-care specialist employed by many spas.

SAUNA, STEAM BATH, AND WHIRLPOOL

Saunas, steam baths, and whirlpools are both therapeutic and relaxing.

Sauna. The dry heat of a sauna can reduce the fat in oil- or fat-based organs such as the liver and gallbladder.

Steam bath. The moist heat of a steam bath is therapeutic to water-based organs such as the kidneys, bladder, and lungs.

Whirlpool. The stimulation of a whirlpool is beneficial to the nervous and lymphatic systems.

MASSAGE

Massage is a therapy that not only reduces emotional and mental stress, but also benefits the body's muscular, lymphatic, nervous, and skeletal systems. For thousands of years, massage has been used for healing; yet it is only recently that studies have shown us its enormous effect. Tiffany Field, Ph.D., director of the Touch Therapy Institute at the University of Miami, has headed studies addressing the psychological, psychiatric, and pediatric uses of massage. Her work has shown that through massage, our immune cells stimulate the nervous system to produce a brain chemical called endorphins that can lower blood pressure and regulate a rapid heartbeat.

ELECTRICAL FREQUENCY AND LASER THERAPY

Electrical and laser therapies are used internationally to safely treat a variety of ailments and to maintain a healthy body. For instance, electrical frequency therapies have been used for more than seventy-five years in sports medicine throughout Europe. These therapies help to reorganize the electrical circuitry of the human body, bringing about a speedy recovery from injury. The realignment of the electrical field of the body also helps to carry away any blockages or maladies. It is well understood that low-frequency lasers can help meet the same goals. Laser therapy helps reorganize cell patterns in human tissues; this acts like a conductor for healing and permits circulatory and electrical order to occur.

High-frequency, electromagnetic energy therapy is now widely used to treat trauma. This painless treatment eliminates edema, absorbs hematoma, and increases blood flow; these biological effects consistently reduce pain and swelling in damaged tissues. Significant acceleration of wound healing has been reported when electromagnetic energy has been applied to burn wounds, plastic surgery sites, finger transplants, and nerve repair. It is also found to relieve pain and inflammation in degenerative and nonarticulated arthritis, and has been successfully used to treat fractured bones (through strapping and plaster casts!)[1] Reports of everything from arthritic pain to tumors have been reduced or eliminated through a series of these noninvasive treatments.

Many complementary health physicians such as naturopathic, osteopathic, and progressive allopathic doctors are now using this technology in their practices. Ask your health-care provider if these therapies would benefit you.

8

Shopping for Your Health

S hopping for the foods you'll need on the Hippocrates diet is easy. You might have to search a bit for a store that has whole foods, but just like your past food shopping trips, you'll make a list, pick up what you need, pay for it, and go home. Nothing's really new here, except the products you're buying. This chapter will steer you through health food stores, mail-order firms, organic foods, supplements, sea vegetables and algae, product labels, and basic food to fill your cupboard.

HEALTH FOOD STORES

As the consumer demand grows, more and more supermarkets are stocking healthful foods. As you read through the recipes in chapter 11, you'll see that many of the ingredients are already in your cabinets or on your grocer's shelves. But other times, you'll need products that are sold only in health food stores. When that's the case, keep the following information in mind.

There are three kinds of health food stores:

1. **Supplement stores:** There are many "health-food" chains cropping up around the world that sell mostly supplements because they have the highest markup for profit. These stores are not really in the health business and shouldn't be visited.
2. **Transitional health food stores:** These stores still dedicate inordinate shelf space to supplements, but also sell some health foods. In a pinch, a savvy shopper can get some of the foods needed on the Hippocrates diet in these stores.
3. **Whole food stores:** Whole food stores typically resemble supermarkets but sell whole, healthy foods. They dedicate much space to organic produce sections and might have their own restaurant and juice bar. They also sell healthful snack foods such as baked crackers, chips with no oil, and raw pickles without vinegar. They'll have products made from living foods such as living sauerkraut, seaweeds, organic grains, beans, seeds, and nuts. Many even have "fast" foods such as instant beans, chickpea patties, whole grain pastas, and soup cups.

Whatever kind of health food store you find in your area, be careful. You can't assume that all the foods they sell are healthful. Many products are packaged with the words "natural," "nature's finest," or "healthy choice," but they are no more good for you than processed foods in the grocery store. The only real difference is in the price—they're much more expensive. Beware of all "natural" canned soups, candies, cakes, pies, chips, ice creams, and frozen "nonmeat" patties. Read the ingredient and nutritional labels carefully. Always check the fat content and the use of additives and preservatives.

MAIL ORDER

Mail-order firms fill a vital shopping need for those who can not conveniently get to health food stores. Many traveling musicians, actors, and salespeople, for example, follow the Hippocrates diet by ordering their food from a mail-order catalog and having it shipped ahead to the hotel where they will be staying. Many of our former Institute guests who spend a lot of time traveling or who are too ill to shop for themselves, do the same.

To find a reputable mail-order food firm, look in the back of natural food magazines such as *Vegetarian Times* or *Organic Gardening*. Start out with a small order to test the quality of the food and the reliability of the firm. You might want to try a few before settling on the one you'll use routinely. And keep current; this is an ever-growing marketplace with more and more new and improved companies ready to offer you what you need to stay conveniently well-nourished.

ORGANIC FOODS

On the Hippocrates diet, most of the foods on your shopping list will be living produce. To get the most from your new diet, make sure the fruits and vegetables you buy are organically grown. Organic foods are grown without the use of chemical fertilizers, herbicides, fungicides, or insecticides. They also are not processed, packaged, transported, or stored with chemicals, artificial additives, or preservatives—nor have they been irradiated. These foods are commonly associated with better flavor and superior nutritional value.

Making a Market for Chemicals

Right up to the mid-1940s, conventional farming was organic. The end of the Second World War found a stockpile of chemicals (designed to maim) sitting in warehouses, taking up space and creating expensive taxable inventories. To solve the problem, a market was created by applying these chemicals to our soil and agricultural plants to kill the bugs and weeds that were destroying some of our food supply.

The initial crop returns were so positive that in the 1950s the world experienced an exponential growth in the use of artificial fertilizers and pesticides, with the United States leading the way. A new economic super industry had been created. In addition, growth promoters, fungicides, herbicides, and insecticides were also used. Sometimes in one growing season, as many as a dozen applications of chemical sprays are used to produce a single crop.

Long-Term Problems

Rather than eliminating the agricultural predators, these chemicals have created an imbalance in our soil, resulting in weakened, poor-quality foods that are more vulnerable to pest infestations than ever before. Rachel Carson predicted as much thirty years ago in her book *Silent Spring*. In more recent years, pesticides' shortcomings have grown harder to ignore as new superbugs become resistant to the chemicals and the beneficial insects are destroyed. In fact, a growing number of agricultural experts now argue that reducing pesticide use would actually decrease pests. When DDT, the first widely used synthetic pesticide, hit the market in 1946, it looked like the silver bullet that would wipe out insect pests forever. Before DDT, American farmers lost about a third of their crops each year to insects, weeds, and disease. Today, with twenty-one thousand pesticide products to choose from and an annual pesticide bill exceeding $4 billion, farmers still lose the same—a one-third share. But the consumer gets more—more harmful chemicals in our shopping baskets.

Pesticides also have a disastrous effect on the nutritional composition of foods. Fifty years ago, wheat grown in Kansas typically had a protein content as high as 14 percent. Today, with the use of chemical fertilizers and monocropping, an all-time low of 8 percent protein in the wheat grown in this grain belt is now the norm. A comparison of an organically grown apple and conventionally grown one shows 300 percent greater Vitamin C and 61 percent greater calcium content in the organic apple.[1]

Not only do conventional fruits and vegetables offer less nutritive value, they pose a medical risk. Some five hundred foreign synthetic chemicals have been found in the human bloodstream. This isn't really surprising considering that the average American consumes trace amounts of chemical residues on their foods amounting to two pounds annually.[2] What is interesting is the correlation that now is being drawn between pesticide consumption and cancer. In one recent study, for example, Mary Wolff, a research scientist at the Mount Sinai Medical Center in New York, found that women with high levels of DDE (a derivative of the pesticide DDT) in their blood were four times as likely to develop breast cancer as women with low levels.[3] I think this and all the similar studies are a wake-up call to food consumers.

How Widespread Is the Problem?

If you don't want to eat chemicals along with your produce, a study released in 1995 by the Agriculture Department's Agricultural Market Service makes it clear that organic foods are your only option. In 1993, the department tested 7,328 fresh apples, bananas, broccoli, celery, carrots, green beans, grapefruit, grapes, lettuce, oranges, peaches, and potatoes. The apples were washed and cored, the bananas were peeled, and the other samples were prepared as if ready to cook or serve.

The scientists discovered 10,329 pesticide residues on the produce, meaning some fruits and vegetables had more than 1 residue. Apples, the most popular fruit, had the highest number of residue detections. Ninety-seven percent of the 654 samples had residues. Celery came next, at 93 percent, and peaches had residues in 91 percent of the sample. The percentages then fell to 79 percent for oranges and potatoes, 75 percent for grapes, and 72 percent for grapefruit. They were followed by green beans, 66 percent; carrots, 65 percent; bananas, 61 percent; lettuce, 51 percent; and broccoli, 25 percent.[4]

Although the EPA says that most pesticide levels found in these foods were below those considered a health risk, this is not reassuring. Some of the pesticide levels were far above the legal limits (especially on imported produce), and the government's approach of regulating each pesticide individually fails to recognize the combined effect on the human body of the different chemicals in one piece of produce. It also ignores the effect on infants and children, who typically eat more fruit and have more sensitive bodies than adults.

The Price of Quality

All of this illustrates why your fruits and vegetables must be organically grown—even if you have to pay a bit more for this guarantee of quality. Organically grown food costs more for several good reasons. The low price we have traditionally paid for our food is partly made possible by the large scale of the agricultural business. Cheap food reflects government subsidy programs and economic support for agriculture, which in most cases is not available to organic farmers. (Fortunately, this situation is starting to change.)

Also, more time is required to grow cover crops and green manures, which provide the needed organic nitrogen. Labor costs are higher for weeding, planting, and harvesting organic crops. The majority of organic growing is still done on medium- and small-sized farms that rely on labor-intensive, nonmechanical activity. It is estimated that there can be a 10 percent to 20 percent higher production cost for organically grown foods and that the end product may cost the consumer from 15 percent to 30 percent to as high as 100 percent more in retail stores.[5]

Organic produce is more expensive, but the bottom line is quality—high quality commands a higher price. And the price will only come down if the supply and demand continue to increase.

Where To Look

Organic produce is getting easier to find as consumer demand rises and a profitable market is created. Organically grown foods traditionally had been found only in natural food stores, natural food cooperatives, health food stores, and farmers' markets. But today, you can find some large supermarkets carrying organic produce. Large grocery chains often carry a limited supply of apples, lettuce, carrots, lemons, and broccoli, for example. Mail-order and natural/organic buying clubs found in the back of health and natural foods magazines are other good sources of organic food supplies.

Check for Certification

Wherever you buy, make sure the food is certified organic. Certification is a voluntary program followed by farmers, ranchers, producers, and processors who agree to strict regulations established by national, international, state, and regional growers' associations. Certification assures the consumer of the authenticity of the products labeled as organically grown, and is very important for increasing the credibility of the organic food movement. Purchasing authentic, certified foods supports the industry and helps ensure that it will endure and grow.

Presently, one-third of the states have legal definitions for organically grown foods. The Organic Foods Production Association of North America (OFPANA) has recommended national standards for organic foods to serve as guidelines as the federal government considers legislation that would authorize the USDA to certify organic foods.

In the meantime, you can purchase food labeled as certified organic with a high degree of reliability. Produce and bulk foods that are not clearly marked as organic with a certification symbol should be assumed to be possibly nonorganic.

What If It's Not Organic?

Sometimes you might not be able to buy organic foods. To help reduce the harmful effects of pesticides, herbicides, fungicides, and fertilizers, keep these tips in mind:

1. Stay away from imported produce. Companies in the U.S. export highly toxic pesticides such as DDT, which are banned for use here. Later, importers turn around and bring in a wide variety of fruits and vegetables from countries that are actively using those poisons on their crops. Then local supermarkets offer them for sale.

2. Wash all fresh fruits and vegetables in water. This will remove some, but not all, of the pesticide residues on the surface. A mild solution of natural dishwashing soap and water may help remove additional surface pesticide residues.
3. Peel produce when appropriate. Peeling the skin from produce will completely remove surface pesticide residues. But residues contained inside the fruit or vegetable will not be eliminated by peeling. (Unfortunately, through peeling, you lose some of the valuable nutrients contained in fresh food.)
4. Grow your own food! Why not try growing your own organic garden? With a small sunny area, you can plant vegetables, or just use large pots or planters. Sprouts are the easiest food to grow; they grow quickly and abundantly in your own kitchen. See chapter 9 for details.

SUPPLEMENTS

The search for supplements may be the most confusing stop on your shopping trip if you aren't sure what you're looking for, or if you are easily swayed by advertising. Many health food stores give more shelf space to supplements than to food! But a 1995 investigation by reporters from *Money* magazine revealed that more than 90 percent of the products sold by health food stores to the investigators were of questionable medical value.

Posing as ordinary consumers, *Money* reporters visited 186 health food stores in thirty-one cities and asked clerks for help. They said they had heard that vitamins and minerals could be beneficial but didn't know what to buy. The clerks sold the reporters an average of $26.13 of products per store, for a total cost of $4,860.18. Nearly all that money was wasted. A full $4,590.42 worth of the products either fell short of the health value requirements of the magazine's health experts or did not carry an expiration date on the label— meaning there was no assurance the product was still effective. In the Los Angeles area alone, supplements pushed by salespeople at five out of six stores had no expiration dates listed.[6]

Let's take a look at the history of supplements to find out how the honorable intent that brought us nutrients in pill form was soon marred by commercial industry.

The History of Herbs and Supplements: The First Generation

Herbs were originally given to the human race by nature. They were used for medicinal purposes when the first human appeared on this planet. For centuries, the formulations were administered only by select individuals—often the spiritual leaders of tribes and societies around the world.

The Second Generation

The second generation of supplements was ushered in by two significant events:

1. Intelligent lay people and practitioners started to understand and use herbs to treat the sick. The leaders of this movement included Arnold Ehret, Paul Bragg, John Tilden, Gaylord Houser, and Jethro Kloss.
2. For the first time, foods and herbs were encapsulated and bottled. Dr. Royal Lee was the first practitioner to prescribe them to patients. The foods and herbs were dried, then ground and put into capsules to preserve their effectiveness. This kind of preparation kept the integrity of the food or herbs intact.

Unfortunately, this generation of supplements fell into decline in the 1930s as the pharmaceutical industry leapt into this increasingly lucrative market.

The Third Generation

The results of encapsulated food and herbs were so positive that "snake oil merchants" began to appear. In this generation, the pharmaceutical industry expanded the market by making synthetic supplements in the laboratory at a fraction of the cost of drying and grinding real foods and herbs. This squeezed out the more expensive natural products.

Individual vitamin and mineral supplements also were introduced. They were extracted from food sources, and then put into tablets or capsules without the whole range of nutrients, called food co-factors, that work symbiotically to allow total absorption of the nutrient into the human cell. Isolated vitamin and mineral products were mass processed with little or no consideration of whole foods; enzymes and oxygen were lost in the processing.

Despite the corruption of quality, the industry continued to grow—from $500 million a year in 1972 to $4.3 billion in 1993.

Are we buying good health with all this money? No. The advertising promises and the high hopes we bring to these little pills and powders might buy us a placebo effect (see chapter 4). But the ingredients the body cells need to thrive are not present. Instead, we're getting color dyes, synthetic binding chemicals, plastic coatings, and test-tube nutrients devoid of the symbiosis found in whole foods.

How do you think your body reacts to this assault? Well, it knows the supplement certainly isn't a food it can use so it calls upon the immune system to launch an attack against the foreign substance. How ironic that millions of people take supplements every day in the hope of building up the immune system without realizing that they are actually wearing down immune cells' strength and resistance.

We now see evidence that the medical community is pulling away from these "miracle" pills. According to the American Diabetes Association, the American Institute of Nutrition, the American Society of Clinical Nutrition, the National Council Against Health Fraud, and the American Medical Association, the practice of taking large doses of vitamin supplements is more than a benign waste of money; it is also dangerous. Megavitamin therapies can lead to nerve damage, internal bleeding, and an array of other health problems. Most recently in 1995, the government's Dietary Guidelines Advisory

Committee argued against routinely using supplements instead of food to get vitamins, minerals, and fibers.

"But," you say, "vitamins are supposed to be good for us!" Understand that 96 percent of the studies conducted on the effectiveness of supplements are underwritten by the companies making and marketing them. When a company invests millions of dollars to develop a product, it is fair to assume that the company will go to any length to "prove" that the supplement works.

In the past, I have never recommended the use of supplements as a dietary complement because I believed that a variety of whole, unprocessed, and unheated foods are intrinsically superior, have a more balanced composition, and can be more fully absorbed. However, now that a new fourth generation of supplements has become available, I am glad to recommend a certain type that complements a living-foods diet.

The Fourth Generation

In the mid-1970s a small group of second generation advocates led a revival of supplements using the best technologies of the third generation. These new products marked the return of whole foods and herbs to the marketplace. Supplements available now respect the wholeness of food that is necessary for effective use by the human body. The processing of these supplements is done at temperatures below 110 degrees to preserves enzymes, oxygen, and important food cofactors; this allows the foods in the supplements to maintain their bioactive quality. Included in this group are the latest generation of green power powders, which use fresh-water, single-cell algae such as chlorella, and Super Blue-Green Algae. These should be used daily when trying to obtain superior and permanent health.

Also in this group are wild herbs and homeopathic remedies. But read the label to find out how they've been prepared. Some extracted herbs and homeopathic products are placed in alcohol. This alters the medicinal structure and at times makes the herbs and homeopathic remedies substantially less effective. In recent years, many herbal and homeopathic manufacturers have found ways to suspend their products in nonintrusive glycerin or water. These properly prepared products are often helpful adjuncts to a living-foods diet. But unlike the whole foods mentioned above, these should be dispensed only by highly trained individuals. They should be taken only for short periods (seldom more than two weeks). Some examples are goldenseal, echinacea, and cats claw. Lighter herbs, such as chamomile, spearmint, and wintergreen, lend themselves to more frequent use in the form of teas. When shopping for supplements, always look for those that are bioactive (made from living, whole foods) and make sure algae and pollens are nonheated. You can write to the Hippocrates Institute for an updated list on the most reputable companies.

We have conducted a series of studies at the institute to determine the benefits of this fourth generation of supplements. We have found that when people are in the process of changing to a healthful lifestyle or in the recovery process from disease, bioactive supplements can contribute up to 30 percent of their physical health gain. But after regulating their systems through lifestyle changes in exercise, attitude, emotion, and food, the majority of subjects gain only 7 percent of the physiological health benefits through this supplementation. Many of us who are healthy choose to continue to use bioactive supplements to gain greater physical endurance and mental acuity but are aware of the limitations.

Sea Vegetables

Be sure to put sea vegetables on your shopping list. The sea is the richest repository of the earth's minerals, and an excellent source of these minerals is readily available to us in sea vegetation. The oceans produce seventeen hundred different species of sea vegetables, but kelp seaweed is the most familiar. More exotic, and perhaps unfamiliar, names such as arame, wakami, nori, and hijiki—as well as the better-known dulse and kelp—are among the sea vegetation that contain twelve key minerals.

Among the health benefits attributed to seaweeds is their ability to stimulate the digestive action of the intestines. Also, the carbohydrates found in seaweed do not elevate the blood-sugar level, so it may be eaten safely by people with blood-sugar problems.

Modern interest in seaweeds started in the West when experiments were carried out in California on cattle that were fed quantities of kelp along with their regular feed. These tests were so successful in eradicating several diseases that further tests were initiated on humans with deficiency diseases. Seaweed was proven a safe and reliable nutritional supplement for correcting certain dietary deficiencies.

Iodine is the only mineral that comes from the sea. The thyroid needs iodine to manufacture a hormone called thyroxin, which aids digestion. Without a sufficient supply of thyroxin, food is burned so slowly that much of it turns to fat. The brain also requires iodine to function; iodine deficiency results in mental sluggishness or varying degrees of retardation. Iodine also kills harmful bacteria in the bloodstream; the blood passes through the thyroid every seventeen minutes for this very purpose. An iodine deficiency is also a contributing factor in enlarged adenoids, fatigue, colds, and infections.

Many other therapeutic minerals are found in abundance in sea plants. Anemia and poor bone and tooth formation can be prevented with adequate intake of cobalt. Healthy blood and fertility rely on zinc and iron. The pituitary uses chlorine and manganese; the adrenals require magnesium; and the pancreas needs nickel and cobalt. Nowhere else can you find such a profuse source of these vital minerals in their natural and most readily usable state as in the wide choice of seaweeds that can be purchased in the better health food stores.

Freshwater Algae

In 1987, after almost two years of study, the Hippocrates Institute added a food group to its diet: single-celled, blue-green and green algae. Now, research results published in the last five years support what we found in our own investigation: algae's nutrition, simple amino acids, enzymes, and genetic coding provide vital elements that are missing from ordinary land-based foods, and it promotes cellular regeneration at the most fundamental (chromosomal) levels.

These simple plants help to convert toxic waste material into harmless substances; provide free radical protection; and supply a balanced profile of vitamins, minerals, and essential and nonessential amino acids. They also supply nutritional enzymes that assist in the digestion of all foods, especially cooked ones. The enzymes break down protein, carbohydrates, and fats.

The Big Three

There are three single-celled algae varieties that I recommend be incorporated into your diet:

Super Blue-Green.   Currently, this algae grows wild and abundantly in only one lake in the world, Klamath Lake in southern Oregon. The main distributor of this algae is a company called Cell Tech. This company revolutionized the algae industry by introducing and perfecting the freeze-drying process, which increases the nutritional and enzyme availability of the algae. This algae comes in two forms, Alpha and Omega. The Alpha regenerates the cells of the body, while the Omega is reported to significantly improve mental facilities.

Spirulina.   Pioneered in North America by Christopher Hill, spirulina is the first blue-green algae to be introduced as a food in the U.S. It grows wild in many locations around the world and is under cultivation to meet current demands. Currently, California and Hawaii lead the world in spirulina production. An immunity builder, spirulina is not easily absorbed by the cell because of its eggshell-type outer wall. We recommend the Hawaiian variety because it is more easily digested.

For years, this algae was dried at a very high temperature. But recently companies that bottle spirulina have adopted the freeze-drying technique, making it a superior product. Make sure the spirulina you buy is freeze-dried.

Chlorella.   Chlorella is a green algae that first gained prominence in Asia, especially Japan. Being high in DNA and RNA, this single-celled algae is noted for enhancing overall body well-being. It has been found to be effective in building one's immune system, normalizing bowel functions, and combating the effects of radiation.

Algae Daily Plan

Different algae plans have been formulated for daily use. Each produces beneficial results; the difference is in the cost. Plan A is least expensive and offers basic benefits; Plan C is most expensive and offers optimum benefits.

Plan A: Cell Tech Omega and Chlorella
Plan B: Cell Tech Omega, Spirulina, and Chlorella
Plan C: Cell Tech Omega and Alpha, and Chlorella

Dosage.   Dosage varies from person to person and from product to product. Read the recommendations on the labels. Initially, reduce the recommended amounts if you want to slow down any possible detoxification reactions, and increase the dosage over several weeks as you feel comfortable. People report that the longer they use algae, the better they feel. (Although the powder form is recommended because it is most efficient, the tablets and capsules are also popular for their convenience.)

When to Take the Algae.   It is best to take algae just before or with your meals. Many people like to sprinkle it on their food. Another option is to take it with your first juice for breakfast.

Improvement.   After the possible detoxification reaction as the algae cleans out the waste materials that may be stored in your body's cells, improvement is usually slow and steady. Within three months, you should be experiencing a boost in energy and improved thinking power.

ANTIOXIDANTS

Antioxidants are compounds believed to help maintain the body's cellular machinery by mopping up dangerous free radicals that can cause cancer. These compounds, which are found naturally in living foods, have been isolated and are now manufactured into synthetic supplements. These little pills have become big business. A very popular antioxidant supplement, beta carotene (which is found naturally in many foods such as carrots, squash, cantaloupes, and peaches), brings in an estimated $75 million each year, according to the director of the National Cancer Institute. But as with other synthetic supplements, the high hopes of those who take these pills don't match the news out of the laboratory.

Two studies funded by the National Cancer Institute and released in 1996 both found that taking a supplement of beta carotene is not equivalent to eating a diet that is rich in fruits and vegetables—in fact, it may be harmful.

The Beta Carotene and Retinol Efficacy Trial (CARET) ended abruptly after four years when investigators told the 18,314 participants to stop taking their supplements. Interim study results indicated that the supplements provided no benefit and might even cause harm. Compared to a group taking a placebo, those taking beta carotene pills had a 28 percent increase in the number of lung cancers and a 17 percent increase in deaths.[7]

In the other trial, the Physicians' Health Study out of Brigham and Woman's Hospital, researchers examined the nutrient's effects in a national sample of 22,071 male physicians for more than twelve years. They found that taking beta carotene conferred no identifiable health benefits or risks. Charles Hennekens, chief of preventive medicine at Brigham and Women's Hospital, echoes my beliefs when he says, "Supplements are no substitute for a healthy diet."[8]

Many researchers now believe it is the combination of antioxidants with other, less-studied components of foods, along with other aspects of a healthful lifestyle, that deliver the health benefits of antioxidants.

PRODUCT LABELS

Because up to 25 percent of your food may be processed foods bought off store shelves, you need to develop the talent of label reading. The face of the package often gives little or misleading information about the value of the food you're buying. So make a habit of reading the ingredient and nutrition labels and following these guidelines:

Ingredients Listing

Usually the shorter the ingredient list, the better:

- Find products that are free of the following known health bandits: meat, fish, chicken, wheat, dairy, eggs, refined sugar (any ingredient ending in "ose"), salt, vinegar, yeast, heated oils, and preservatives.
- Eliminate or limit the use of products that contain refined sugar substitutes such as barley malt, brown rice syrup, date sugar, honey, and Succanat (raw sugar). Substitute with stevia.
- Tofu and most other soybean products are difficult to digest; use them sparingly. They are a hard-to-utilize source of healthful protein.
- Added vitamins and minerals are of questionable value at best. We think of them as possible agents for disease and immune dysfunction. Avoid them when possible.

Nutritional Information

Comparison shopping is a must for carbohydrates, fats, and protein. New labeling regulations make it relatively easy to evaluate the content of these three food factors. Follow these suggestions for a one-ounce (twenty-eight gram) serving:

- Fat and protein per serving should be less than three grams (10 percent)—the lower, the better.
- The carbohydrate grams should be at least five times greater than the total of both the fat and protein grams. For example, if the label says there are two grams of fat and three grams of protein in a single serving, you'll want to see at least fifteen grams of carbohydrates.
- When comparing labels, look for the lower percentage of saturated fat. Saturated fat has been identified as a factor in coronary disease and some cancers.

SHOPPING FOR RECREATIONAL FOODS

Recreational foods are the ones that entertain the emotions and the memory more than nutritional needs. The following items are not optimal foods, but are improvements on items normally consumed. Most of these items have appeared on the shelves in health food stores over the years, but are still not generally available in conventional supermarkets. These items should make up 10 percent or less of your daily diet. *Starred items are the best choices in the category.*

FROZEN AND REFRIGERATED FOODS

Look for items with no dairy, wheat, added oil, salt, or sugar (including honey, barley, corn or rice syrups, fructose, sucrose, maltose).

Ice Cream/Fruit Bars

organic sorbet*
fruit bars
fruit sticks
rice "ice cream"

Hamburgers/Hot Dogs

tempeh
soy dogs
tofu burgers
bean patties

Pizza

rice crust pizza (with soy cheese)

Cheese Substitute

mochi, plain (in deli section)
lowfat soy cheese

Frozen Vegetables

frozen organic vegetables

Wheat Bagel Substitutes

spelt, rye, or quinoa bagels

DRY GOODS

Look to eliminate fat, oil, wheat, dairy, eggs, salt, and hidden sugar.

Breads

essene rye
corn tortilla
100 percent sour
    dough spelt, rye,
    and kumit

Cereals

cream of rye
puffed corn
puffed millet*
buckwheat
teff

Peanut Butter Substitutes

raw almond butter
raw sunflower butter
raw tahini

Chips/Snacks

baked sweet potato chips
baked tortilla chips
air popped popcorn*
baked apple chips
baked carrot chips

Milk Substitutes

Amazake (rice drink)
rice milk beverage
white almond beverage

Crackers/Crisps

brown rice snaps
rice cakes (plain is best)

Sugar/Honey Substitutes

maple syrup (65 percent sugar)
stevia *

Quick Dips

lowfat refried beans *
quick hummus

Salt Substitute

Braggs Aminos

Flour

quinoa flour
corn flour
rye flour
spelt flour
teff flour*
amaranth flour

Butter Substitutes

canola oil
flaxseed oil
olive oil (Carothers brand is best)
sesame oil
nonhydrogenated lowfat spread

Coffee Substitutes

herb teas (caffeine-free)
Yannoh organic grain
    coffee substitute

Chocolate

carob powder

Soft Drink

fruit juice diluted with
    water

MAKE YOUR LIST

When you read through the recipes in chapter 11, pick out a few you'd like to experiment with, jot down the ingredients, and go shopping! It's fun to find new stores and products. It's a creative experience that breaks up the boring routine of buying and eating the same foods day after day. Enjoy your venture into healthy and living foods.

9

In the Kitchen with Living Foods

Some of the foods required in the Hippocrates diet can be prepared in your own kitchen. This chapter will discuss germinating and sprouting, the use of grasses and leafy green vegetables, the value of juicing, and the exciting use of some dehydrated and fermented foods.

GERMINATING AND SPROUTING

Many ancient cultures knew the value of germinating and sprouting grains, seeds, legumes, and nuts. Today, more and more information is being compiled on the amazing nutritional value of sprouting:

- Researchers at Purdue University found that bean sprouts contain extraordinarily high levels of good-quality protein. Mung bean sprouts, for example, contain more than 25 percent of their calories as protein, which is a higher proportion than in T-bone steak. And soybean sprouts have an even greater percentage. Because of their high levels of amino acids (the building blocks of protein), vitamins, and minerals, sprouts are considered to be one of the most perfect foods known to man.

- Dr. P. R. Burkholder of Yale University showed that when oats are sprouted, the vitamin B2 (riboflavin) content increases by 1,300 percent, vitamin B6 (pyridoxine) by 500 percent, and folic acid by 600 percent. Because of these enormous increases over the vitamin content of dried grains and seeds, Dr. Burkholder recommended the wide-scale use of sprouts as food in the West.
- Dr. C. McCay of the Cornell University School of Nutrition was hired by the U.S. government during the Second World War to find suitable protein substitutes for meat, poultry and dairy foods because of expected wartime shortages. After months of research, Dr. McCay concluded that sprouted beans would fill the need quite well. He wrote several articles, including instructions and recipes that were available through the U.S. Government Printing Office, but since the protein shortages never came, the campaign to educate Americans about the nutritional value of sprouts was dropped.
- Research in the late 1970s at the University of Puget Sound found that six cups of sprouted lentils contain the full recommended daily allowance of protein (about 60 grams) in a fully digestible form. Scientists concluded that lentil sprouts could provide a significant portion of daily protein needs in a safe and inexpensive form.

Living foods that are germinated and sprouted give us the most concentrated natural sources of vitamins, minerals, enzymes, and amino acids (proteins in a digestible form). They also provide abundant enzymes and bioelectrical energy, boosting their daily desirability. Pound for pound, lentils and other bean sprouts contain as much protein as red meat, yet are totally digestible and have none of the fat, cholesterol, hormones, or antibiotics found in most present-day meats.

Germination

Germination results when seeds, grains, legumes, and nuts are soaked in water for a period of time. Water removes certain metabolic inhibitors that protect the seed from bacterial invasion and preserve it during its dormant state. During germination, the seed springs into life, increasing its nutritional value and digestibility. Inherent enzyme inhibitors, phytates (natural insecticides), and oxalates (protective shields that prevent oxygen from penetrating) present in every seed, nut, bean, and grain, are removed and predigestion occurs. In this predigestion stage, starches are converted into simple sugars, proteins are broken down into amino acids, fats are converted into soluble fatty acids, and vitamins are created. Germination is used to make many of the seed and nut sauces suggested in recipes in chapter 11. It is also the first step in sprouting. But even if you plan to cook your grains or beans, you should germinate them first. (Due to their high oil content, do not ever cook seeds or nuts.)

Germinating a seed, nut, grain, or legume is beautifully simple (see Figure 9-1). Basically, all that is needed is a jar, seeds, water, light and oxygen. Soak the seeds or nuts the required time in room-temperature, with pure water. Then pour off the cloudy water (save it to water houseplants, which thrive on it), then rinse well to remove all inhibitors before food preparation. The seeds or nuts are now ready to be used.

The soaking time varies according to the size of the seed or nut. All small seeds such as alfalfa, radish, red clover, sesame, cabbage, and mustard can be soaked from four to six hours. Slightly larger seeds such as wheat, barley, fenugreek, buckwheat, and sunflower should be soaked for six to eight hours. Larger nuts and beans such as almonds, filberts, Brazil nuts, pintos, and chickpeas should be soaked for ten to twelve hours. However, climate, season, and temperature play a significant role; in warmer environments, soaking time is reduced.

Figure 9-1 Seeds, nuts, grains, and legumes sprouting method.

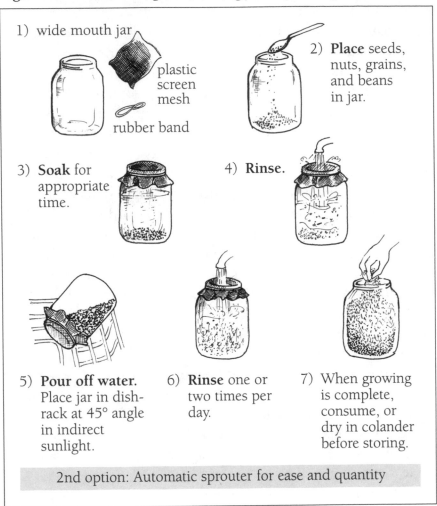

1) wide mouth jar

plastic
screen
mesh

rubber band

2) **Place** seeds, nuts, grains, and beans in jar.

3) **Soak** for appropriate time.

4) **Rinse.**

5) **Pour off water.** Place jar in dish-rack at 45° angle in indirect sunlight.

6) **Rinse** one or two times per day.

7) When growing is complete, consume, or dry in colander before storing.

2nd option: Automatic sprouter for ease and quantity

Sprouting

Sprouting carries the germinating process one step further, resulting in a variety of living foods, such as small alfalfa, clover, and radish sprouts, as well as sprouts from sunflower seeds and buckwheat seeds. (Later in this chapter you'll learn how to grow the latter two on trays.)

Sprouts can be bought in many supermarkets, but to increase your supply, improve the quality, add variety, and reduce the cost, you can grow them yourself in just a few simple steps:

To begin, you will need wide-mouth jars, plastic screen mesh, and a rubber band to secure the mesh to the top of the jar, and, of course, the seeds, nuts, grains, or beans. (Business people and others who are often away from home will find automatic sprouters useful; when traveling, sprouting can be done in sprouting bags.)

First pour one cup of seeds, nuts, grains, or beans into a jar. Cover with plenty of water. Put the mesh over the top of the jar and secure with the rubber band. Place the jar out of direct sunlight and let the products soak in room-temperature water for the appropriate time (see the Hippocrates Sprouting Chart on page 170). Pour off the water and rinse well. Turn the jar upside-down and let it drain. (Use a dish drainer to hold the jar at an angle.) From this point until they are stored, the seeds should stay well drained yet moist, get adequate air, and be kept warm in a dark or semidark location during the sprouting stages. Rinse the sprouts morning and evening to keep them from drying out. Rinse them more frequently in dry warmer climates when the sprouts grow more quickly and so are more prone to spoil.

Between rinsings, keep the jars upside down in a dish drainer at a forty-five-degree angle to allow for drainage and circulation. When they are ready, you will want to remove the hulls of seeds such as alfalfa, fenugreek, cabbage, mung, adzuki, and radish. (Others such as the grains, hulled sunflower seeds, sesame seeds, lentils, and chick-peas can be eaten as they are.) To remove hulls, place the sprouts in the sink or a large pan and fill with rushing water. Carefully shake the sprouts to loosen the hulls and when they rise to the top, brush the hulls aside. Next, carefully lift the soaking sprouts out of the water so as not to disturb any hulls that are floating along the side or have sunk to the bottom. Place the hulled sprouts in a colander to drain.

Allow the cleaned sprouts to dry before putting them in the refrigerator. To store sprouts in the refrigerator, place them in glass or plastic containers lined with paper towels to absorb excess moisture. Once refrigerated, rinse and drain the sprouts every three to four days to increase the "expiration date" from several days to several weeks. (But remember: the sooner you eat them, the richer they are in nutrients.)

Special Instructions

- To harvest nuts, simply pour off the soak water, rinse the nuts, and replace them in fresh water. For storage, place nuts in the refrigerator in fresh water.
- Small seeds such as alfalfa increase in weight and volume after sprouting, so don't overfill the jar at the beginning.
- The chlorophyll content of the small vegetable seeds can be increased. After they develop their first two leaves, place the sprouts in abundant, indirect sunlight for twelve to twenty-four hours to green them up.

MUNG AND ADZUKI GROWING

Follow this process for growing sweet, juicy mung bean and adzuki sprouts:

Soaking.   Very warm (130 to 140 degrees F.) soak water is the key to developing a sweet sprout. If possible, change the soak water several times during the soaking process, or keep the soaking seeds in a very warm location.

Sprouting.   The secret to long, straight, and juicy sprouts is to grow them under pressure in a warm, dark place. One way to do this is to grow them in a stainless steel colander with a heavy plate on top of them. You might think this will squash them, but it doesn't; they grow larger and stronger.

Figure 9-2 Mung and adzuki sprouting method.

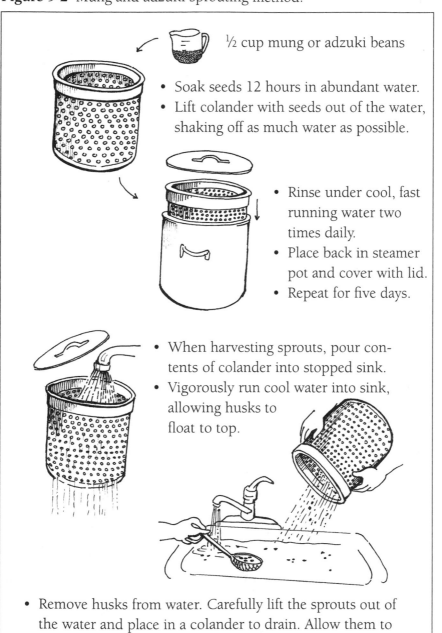

½ cup mung or adzuki beans

- Soak seeds 12 hours in abundant water.
- Lift colander with seeds out of the water, shaking off as much water as possible.

- Rinse under cool, fast running water two times daily.
- Place back in steamer pot and cover with lid.
- Repeat for five days.

- When harvesting sprouts, pour contents of colander into stopped sink.
- Vigorously run cool water into sink, allowing husks to float to top.

- Remove husks from water. Carefully lift the sprouts out of the water and place in a colander to drain. Allow them to dry before eating or placing in the refrigerator.

Hippocrates Sprouting Chart

Seed Type	Dry Measure	Soaking Time	Sprouting Time	Yield	Length at Harvest
HULLED SEEDS					
Buckwheat	1 cup	6 hrs.	24 hrs.	2 cups	⅛"
Pumpkin	1 cup	4 hrs.	24 hrs.	2 cups	⅛"
Sesame	1 cup	4 hrs.	12 hrs.	1½ cups	⅛"
Sunflower	1 cup	6 hrs.	24 hrs.	2 cups	¼–½"

NUTRITIONAL AND HEALTH BENEFITS
Buckwheat: lecithin
Pumpkin: hair and skin
Sesame: calcium
Sunflower: protein and energy

Seed Type	Dry Measure	Soaking Time	Sprouting Time	Yield	Length at Harvest
SMALL GRAINS (ALKALIZING GRAINS)					
Amaranth	1 cup	3 hrs.	24 hrs.	3 cups	⅛"
Millet	1 cup	5 hrs.	12 hrs.	3 cups	0–⅛"
Quinoa	1 cup	3 hrs.	24 hrs.	3 cups	¼"
Teff	1 cup	3 hrs.	24 hrs.	3 cups	⅛"

NUTRITIONAL AND HEALTH BENEFITS
Amaranth: bone strengthening
Millet: strength and muscle
Quinoa: strength and energy
Teff: blood and respiration

Seed Type	Dry Measure	Soaking Time	Sprouting Time	Yield	Length at Harvest
LARGE GRAINS (MORE ACID-FORMING GRAINS)					
Barley	1 cup	6 hrs.	12 hrs.	2½ cups	0"
Corn	1 cup	12 hrs.	36 hrs.	4 cups	½"
Rye	1 cup	6 hrs.	36 hrs.	3 cups	¼"
Spelt	1 cup	6 hrs.	36 hrs.	3 cups	¼"
Triticale	1 cup	6 hrs.	36 hrs.	3 cups	¼"
Wheat	1 cup	6 hrs.	36 hrs.	3 cups	¼"

Nutritional and Health Benefits

Barley: ventricles and heart
Corn: calcium and energy
Rye: digestion and roughage
Spelt: vitamins and minerals
Triticale: calcium, vitamins, and minerals
Wheat: vitamins and minerals

Beans and Legumes

Adzuki	½ cup	12 hrs.	5 days	4 cups	1"
(grow under pressure)					
Chickpeas	1 cup	12 hrs.	3 days	4 cups	1"
Lentils	¾ cup	8 hrs.	3 days	4 cups	1"
Green peas	1½ cups	8 hrs.	3 days	4 cups	1"
Lima	2 cups	12 hrs.	12 hrs.	4 cups	0"
Mung	⅓ cup	8 hrs.	5 days	4 cups	2"
(grow under pressure)					
Northern white	1½ cups	12 hrs.	12 hrs.	4 cups	0"
Pinto	1 cup	12 hrs.	3 days	4 cups	1"

Nutritional and Health Benefits

Adzuki: minerals and renal benefits
Chickpeas: protein and energy
Lentils: teeth and strength
Green peas: blood and organs
Lima: nails and eyes
Mung: minerals and bladder benefits
Northern white: energy and liver
Pinto: energy and spine

Small Vegetables

Alfalfa	3 tbls.	5 hrs.	5 days	4 cups	2"
Cabbage	3 tbls.	5 hrs.	5 days	4 cups	1½"

Clover	3 tbls.	5 hrs.	5 days	4 cups	2"
Fenugreek	¼ cup	6 hrs.	5 days	4 cups	2"
Garlic	¼ cup	5 hrs.	5 days	3 cups	1"
Kale	¼ cup	5 hrs.	5 days	4 cups	1"
Mustard	3 tbls.	5 hrs.	5 days	4 cups	1½"
Onion	¼ cup	5 hrs.	5 days	3 cups	1½"
Radish	3 tbls.	6 hrs.	5 days	4 cups	2"
Turnip	3 tbls.	6 hrs.	4 days	4 cups	1½"

NUTRITIONAL AND HEALTH BENEFITS

Alfalfa: blood and heart

Cabbage: intestine and stomach

Clover: capillaries and blood

Fenugreek: dissolves mucus and deposits

Garlic: heart and cholesterol

Kale: bowel

Mustard: stomach and gallbladder

Onion: blood and circulation

Radish: lymph and hormones

Turnip: colon and intestine

Note: These are just a few from among thousands of seeds, nuts, grains, and beans to sprout.

GRASS JUICE

Wheatgrass, spelt grass, kumit grass, and barley grass are vital parts of the Hippocrates diet that can be prepared in your kitchen. These grasses are used primarily for making therapeutic juice, but they have other uses as well. The blades of the grass can be chewed, the juice extracted in the mouth, and the pulp discarded (not swallowed). This will freshen stale breath or relieve sore throats. The grasses can also be chewed to relieve sore teeth and gums. The juice can be applied to burns, cuts, rashes, poison ivy, and insect bites; or it can be soaked up in a lump of semi-dried grass and placed in a bandage to help heal boils, open sores, external ulcers, tumors, and other skin problems.

Wheatgrass is one of nature's richest sources of vitamins A and C. It contains all the known minerals your body needs such as calcium, iron, magnesium, phosphorous, potassium, sodium, sulfur, cobalt, and zinc, as well as all essential amino acids, which makes it a complete protein. It's also rich in the B vitamins, especially B-17 (more commonly known as laetrile), which is said to selectively destroy cancer cells without affecting normal cells. Wheatgrass juice also aids digestion and can be used to help relieve many internal pains. It has been used to treat peptic ulcer and ulcerative colitis.

Decades of research and application at the institute have found that this plant gets its miraculous powers from the massive amounts of vitamin-rich chlorophyll it contains. When scientists examined wheatgrass, they found that chlorophyll makes up a large percentage of the grass' composition after the water is extracted. Wheatgrass is very similar to the chemical molecular structure of human red blood cells, enhancing the blood's capacity to carry oxygen to every cell of the body. This amazing natural substance also produces an environment that suppresses bacterial growth in the body and counteracts toxins that have been ingested. Nature uses the chlorophyll in wheatgrass as a body cleanser, rebuilder, and neutralizer of the toxins that accumulate in our bodies and poison our systems. The accumulations of these toxins contribute to degenerative diseases such as arthritis, diabetes, and heart disease. Dr. G. H. Erp-Thomas, scientist and soil expert, isolated more than one hundred elements from fresh wheatgrass and concluded that it is a complete food.[1] Fifteen pounds of fresh wheatgrass is equivalent in nutritional value to 350 pounds of the choicest vegetables.

Wheatgrass and Graingrass Preparation

To prepare wheatgrass or other graingrass in your kitchen, purchase organic, whole winter-wheat or other hard-grain kernels at your local

Figure 9-3 Sprouting at home.

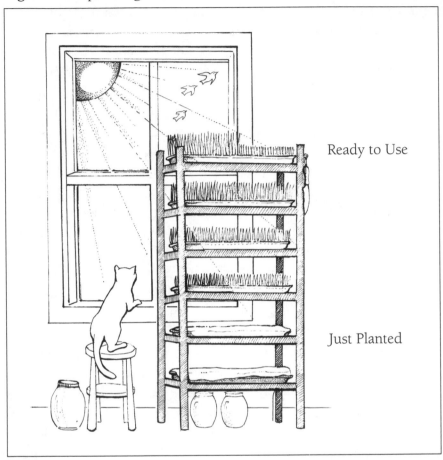

Ready to Use

Just Planted

health food store. Obtain several trays a half inch deep and measuring 14 by 18 inches. (We use cafeteria trays, which can be purchased from restaurant supply stores.) The trays hold the soil and seeds; you can use another as a cover to hold in the moisture, or you can use black plastic. If you want to have one tray of wheatgrass available to use every day, you'll need a total of eight trays in all (sixteen if you want to use trays as covers). You'll also need organic soil from a nursery (or dig it up from a publicly-owned forest if allowed) combined with 50 percent peat moss. (As you progress, you can produce the highest quality compost from discarded root mats and vegetable table scraps.)

To plant wheatgrass, soak one cup of whole winter-wheat seeds from six to twelve hours in a lot of water, and then sprout for another twelve hours with the jar upside down in a dish drainer. In warm weather, rinse at least two times to prevent drying out.

Spread a one-inch layer of soil in a tray and make drainage troughs or a gutter along the four sides. Spread the germinated seeds evenly over the tray, being careful not to let them spill in the trough. Also, try not to let the seeds pile on top of one another. Then water thoroughly, but do not overwater. (You can tell if you have over-watered if you see water standing in the gutter.) Next, place another tray or black plastic over the seeds and leave for three days, or until the sprouts start pushing up the cover. Uncover, water thoroughly, and place in a bright spot but not in direct sunlight. Water once a day along the trough, and sprinkle the soil and growing sprouts. Your plants will be mature enough to use in about seven days, depending on weather and climate. Harvest by cutting the grass at the soil line with a sharp knife or scissors.

After harvesting, refrigerate the grass to prevent complete deterioration. But keep a continual supply of wheatgrass growing, because these sprouts lose most of their potency after one week. You may also purchase an automatic sprouter and avoid the soil growing and effort.

TRAY GREENS

Besides wheatgrass and graingrass, the green sprouts of sunflower and buckwheat seeds are also integral to the Hippocrates diet. These are sprouted then planted in soil on trays similar to wheatgrass. Sunflower greens contain a full spectrum of amino acids (the building blocks of protein) and supply vitamin D without the problems inherent in dairy sources. These baby greens contain an abundance of sun energy and chlorophyll, and are considered a complete food. Buckwheat lettuce is very high in bioactive lecithin and helps eliminate deposits on arterial walls. It is also an excellent source of chlorophyll and contains good amounts of B-vitamins such as riboflavin (the red you see in the stems) and rutin (food for the

Figure 9-4 Three types of tray greens.

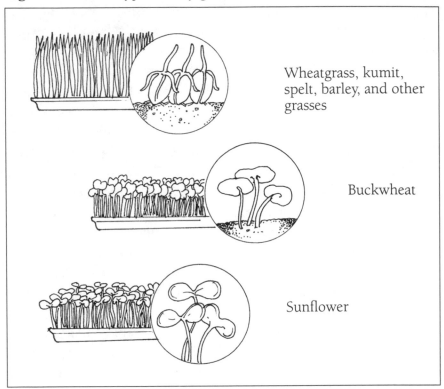

Wheatgrass, kumit, spelt, barley, and other grasses

Buckwheat

Sunflower

brain). These tray sprouts are eaten in salads shortly after harvesting and are juiced for green drinks (see below).

Tray Preparation for Green Sprouts

The procedure for growing tray-grown sprouts of sunflower and buckwheat is similar to the wheatgrass procedure. Be sure to buy organically grown or biologically grown seeds with their hulls left on.

For each tray, begin by soaking the seeds in large jars. Use 1½ cups sunflower seeds and fill the jar with 4 cups water or use 1½ cups dry buckwheat seeds in 2 cups water. Soak for eight hours, then drain the seeds and allow them to sprout for twelve hours. Plant and harvest these germinated seeds following the tray procedure outlined on page 173 for wheatgrass.

TROUBLE-SHOOTING

If your sprouts and tray greens do not grow into healthy greens, check this trouble-shooting list for possible reasons:

Seeds do not sprout
- You soaked the seeds too long.
- The seeds were old and dead to start with.

Seeds sprouted, but did not grow well
- The soil was not kept moist.
- The soil was kept too moist.
- The quality of the soil might have been poor.

Mold is plentiful
The seeds that do not sprout will naturally mold. Problem areas may be:
- The trays were kept too moist, or the seeds were planted too close together and could not breathe. Increase air circulation with a fan or use an Alpine (oxygen-generating) air purifier to reduce mold.
- The humidity was too high. Again, a fan and dehumidifier will help. Sometimes, covering the seeds and soil with plastic for the first three days creates the problem; try growing without it. If the problem still persists, soak your seeds in a mixture of 2 tablespoons hydrogen peroxide in a gallon of water.

JUICING

Fresh juices are another key to the Hippocrates Program. The extracted juices from fresh vegetables, some fruits, sprouts, and tray-grown green sprouts allow us to get all the benefits of their outstanding nutritional qualities in an easily assimilated form. Juices are digested immediately and begin cleansing and healing long before the same whole foods can begin to work. In addition, whole foods use up valuable energy because of the prolonged digestion process.

Juicing is not the same thing as blending or even liquefying. A blender makes a fruit or vegetable appear liquefied, but a juicer extracts only the liquid, leaving the cellulose or fiber behind. At the institute, we use several juicers for preparing fresh juices. The non-centrifugal Champion-type juicers are excellent machines, ideal for making a variety of juices. Also preferred are pressure-press or auger-press juicers; these are low speed machines that press the juice out of the more fibrous sprouts, greens, and grass—a job that the high speed machines can not do efficiently.

All fresh juices should be consumed as soon as possible, before they lose their natural potency. Grass juices, in particular, are not stable and tend to go bad quickly; it's best to drink your grass juice immediately or within fifteen minutes after preparation.

Be advised that wheatgrass is a powerful cleanser, and it may cause nausea in some people soon after ingestion. This is merely a reaction to the release of toxins within the system. Start with small quantities, one ounce or so, and then each day gradually increase the intake to three or four ounces. (Wheatgrass juice is also used as part of a sound colon-cleansing program by implanting the juice directly into the colon as explained in chapter 7.)

Green Drinks

Green drinks are vital to health and well-being. These are made from juiced sunflower and buckwheat sprouts and vegetables such as cucumbers, celery, parsley, watercress, sweet red peppers, and kale. All are juiced in the slow-turning press juicers. What gives these drinks their healing qualities is that they are made almost entirely from the indoor tray-grown sprouts. These are the most alive of the living foods and the other vegetables are added merely for flavor. I suggest drinking at least two twelve-ounce glasses of green drink per day. These drinks are an exceptional source of chlorophyll. They supply from one-third to one-half of the protein needed by the average adult each day. And they have a cleansing and alkalinizing effect upon the body.

Drink green drinks within fifteen minutes of preparation to gain the oxygen, enzymes, and nutrients that rapidly diminish with time. You can refrigerate these drinks, but their impact will be dramatically reduced.

DEHYDRATED FOODS

Dehydration is a good bridge between cooked and raw foods. Drying fruits, vegetables, nut-and-seed mixtures with readily available home dehydrators opens another door to a whole world of healthy, nutritious, and delicious eating. While some vitamin and enzyme breakdown occurs during dehydration, it is still much preferred to cooking.

When preparing a menu of dehydrated foods, use fruits sparingly. While small amounts of fruit in the daily diet are usually beneficial, a high amount of fruit in your diet makes it too rich in sugar and aggravating to certain illnesses, such as high or low blood sugar, vaginal yeast infections, *Candida albicans,* cancer, and viral problems. Therefore, when dehydrating, use more vegetables and less fruit. If you are ill, avoid dried fruits completely.

FERMENTED FOODS

Fermented foods may be part of your Hippocrates diet, but use sparingly. For many years, we advocated a wide variety of fermented foods and drinks for all people. Certain important and friendly bacteria grow during the fermentation process. These bacilli encourage healthy intestinal fauna and regulate bowel movements. But over the years, we noticed that they sometimes caused adverse reactions. Fermented drinks and fermented seed cheeses and nut loaves were found occasionally to harbor unfriendly bacteria. Fermented foods were legitimate and desirable for many people's diets, but some found many of these foods irritating. Now we feel that the health benefits of fermentation are best derived from only the occasional use of raw sauerkraut. We also suggest that people with fungal, mold, yeast, or bacterial infections should avoid sauerkraut until they are well.

KITCHEN SUPPLIES

Before you browse through chapter 11 and select your favorite recipes, take a moment to think about the kitchen supplies you'll need to stay on the Hippocrates diet. A well-stocked kitchen should have the following items:

- a juicer (noncentrifugal Champion-type, or pressure- or auger-press juicers)
- a dehydrator
- a blender or food processor
- sharp knives
- a good cutting board

You can find these items at your local health food store and in some appliance stores.

10

Eating in the Real World

Once you are ready and determined to adopt the Hippocrates Health Program, a few practical questions arise:

- How do I prepare food for my family?
- What should I do when I'm invited to a friend's house?
- Can I eat in restaurants?
- What should I do when I travel?

FAMILY FOOD PREPARATION

As you begin your new health program, do not try to convince everyone in your family that you have discovered the best way of eating and try to convert them all. Instead, quietly make the changes in your life that you are committed to for your own health and bring your family into the program in small steps each day:

1. Remove the most dangerous foods from your kitchen. These include foods high in complex fats and protein, sugar, salt, and chemical additives (including isolated vitamins and mineral supplements). Also, get rid of alcohol and vinegar. Replace these with the "healthier" products now available in healthmarkets. Remember to take small steps at first. Instead of Fruit Loops, try organic grain cereal. Instead of ice cream, try frozen fruit bars.

2. Don't stock up on the unhealthy foods that your family is unwilling to do without. Let a few days go by before you replenish the cabinet. As you wean them from these items, increase the number of healthier bioactive foods available to them. The key is not to make them feel deprived, but rather to introduce them to healthier alternatives gradually. Slowly replace refined grain products with whole grain products; dairy milks, cheeses, and yogurts with low-fat almond, rice, and soy varieties; white potatoes with sweet potatoes and yams; and highly sugared desserts with fresh fruit cocktails or Carob Banana Ice-Bars (see chapter 11 for recipes).

3. Replace more hazardous methods of cooking, such as microwaving and frying, with dehydrating, steaming, and baking.

4. Make the centerpiece of every dinner a mixed salad of sprouts and various in-season vegetables (especially the green leafy ones).

5. Experiment with making salad dressings and sauces using avocado, soaked nuts, or sprouted beans as the base (see chapter 11 for recipes).

6. Prepare at least one recipe from this book for yourself at every meal. (This should add no more than 15 minutes to your preparation time.) Let your family see these foods and offer them a taste.

FRIENDS

As with your family, the trick to eating with your friends is to do what's best for you without insulting or imposing on others.

1. Knowing that food is going to be at most social engagements, eat before you go to satisfy your appetite. This will make you

less inclined to overindulge in fattening and unhealthy foods while visiting.

2. Let your friends know that you have been placed on a diet that is low in complex fats and proteins, salt, refined sugars, dairy, and wheat products. Explain to them that the program follows the latest guidelines of major medical universities and the U.S. government for reducing chronic disease. If they truly are your friends, they will understand; perhaps they even might show an interest in knowing more.

3. Offer to bring a dish (perhaps a salad or your favorite appetizer) when you go to a friend's home. This guarantees you something to eat if nothing else to your liking is served.

4. Do not refuse to eat a bite or two at the expense of offending (or even losing) a friend. Most people are happy if you only taste what they have made for you, but they may be put off if you refuse to sample even a morsel. Use your best judgment.

5. Locate vegetarian groups in your area as a new way to meet people with a common goal. Your local health food store is an excellent resource for this. These groups usually sponsor monthly get-togethers for food, fun, and education.

RESTAURANTS

Here's an area that will take some exploring on your part. Unless you can find restaurants that serve dishes made with organically grown foods, it's best to limit your outings to twice a month. When you locate restaurants that serve food free of pesticides and preservatives, eat there often, and tell your friends about the great food! Here are a few tips for dining out:

1. It's always a good idea to eat a little before you go out so you're not tempted to eat everything in sight.

2. Most restaurants do offer some type of salad on the menu. The key is to find the ones that offer the largest variety of raw vegetables, especially sprouts, with the least amount of pesticides.

3. Look through the phone book and newspapers for places that offer high-quality vegetarian choices, even if most of the menu items are cooked. Make phone calls to restaurant managers to share your dietary concerns on chemicals (pesticides) on food, heated oils and proteins, excess fat, processed sugar, and preservatives such as salt and MSG. You may be pleasantly surprised at their positive response.

4. Before going to a restaurant, call first to find out if a special meal can be prepared. Ask if they'll make a salad of raw vegetables. Most better restaurants are more than happy to accommodate you.

5. Always be ready to make a suggestion when deciding where to go to eat. It's easy for the omnivores (people who eat anything put on a plate in front of them) to find something to their liking, even in a vegetarian restaurant.

6. Take a good all-purpose digestive enzyme with every meal when you eat out or eat cooked foods. Enzyme supplements (such as the ones developed at the Hippocrates Health Institute) contain traces of sea algae, fresh water algae, and land-based nutritional grasses. They help break down fat, protein, and carbohydrates. They also introduce bioactive foods into the digestive tract to aid nutrient absorption.

7. The better traditional restaurant choices are those that specialize in Asian (Japanese, Chinese, Thai), Middle Eastern (Lebanese, Egyptian, Turkish), Greek, and Mexican cuisines. The majority of traditional American and European continental restaurants have little to offer to Hippocrates advocates.

TRAVELING

Traveling puts most of us in unfamiliar territory and, therefore, makes it difficult to stay on the Hippocrates diet. But it can be done with some advance thinking:

1. Always take your algae products and all-purpose digestive enzymes with you to provide high-octane nutrition.

2. When flying, be sure to ask your airline for a vegetarian meal at the time you purchase your ticket. Call twenty-four hours before departure to confirm your request. If a vegetarian meal is not available, bring your own sprout salad or ripe fruit. This can also be done when traveling by train.
3. When traveling by car or bus, bring a cooler loaded with fresh vegetables and fruit. If you are on the road for days, replenish your stock with the best produce you can find. Use the local phone books to help you locate organic produce markets.
4. When traveling to foreign countries, especially the Third World, bring nuts and seeds and soak or sprout them along the way. Also, carry some (food-grade) hydrogen peroxide to wash pesticide residues and parasites from your vegetables and fruits. If this is not available, use vinegar as a substitute.

It will take some time to settle into your healthier lifestyle and sometimes you'll need to employ some flexible thinking and creative solutions. But it can be done. I travel all over the world; I eat in many restaurants every year; I visit scores of people in their homes; and yet I strictly adhere to the Hippocrates diet. Combine the tips in this chapter with your own ingenuity and you'll find that your new diet will not upset your family or ever cramp your social or travel plans.

11

Time to Eat: Living-Foods Recipes

I have kept to a diet of living foods for more than two decades, and I find it more exciting each day as my family's health increases. Along with my wife, children, and my staff at the institute, I am always looking for new ways to enjoy foods that are enzyme- and oxygen-rich, while keeping in mind the rules of food combining. The recipes that follow are a sampling from my family's recipe box that will give you a good idea of how you, too, can put together living foods in ways that are wholesome, satisfying, and truly delicious. (Although not specified, all ingredients should be organically grown.)

The ingredient glossary at the end of this book defines ingredients you may not be familiar with. *An asterisk after an ingredient in a recipe means it is included in the glossary.*

I've also included a sample one-week meal plan in this chapter. Give these meals a try, and don't hesitate to be creative by altering any recipe to suit your taste.

If you come up with an especially good, original living-foods recipe, I'd love to hear about it. If the chefs at the Hippocrates Health Institute give your creation a thumbs up, we'll name the dish after you and serve it with much fanfare to our guests.

Send your recipes to:

Recipes
The Hippocrates Health Institute
1443 Palmdale Court
West Palm Beach, FL 33411

Hors D'oeuvres

GUACAMOLE

2 red bell peppers
1 zucchini
2 tablespoons kelp*
2 avocados
½ teaspoon powdered raw
   cayenne pepper

3 tablespoons minced onion
1 teaspoon chopped parsley
1 teaspoon paprika
1 teaspoon chopped basil

Place 1 of the red bell peppers, ½ of the zucchini, and the kelp in a blender, and blend until smooth. Transfer to a bowl.

Mash the avocados into the red bell pepper mixture. Stir in the remaining ingredients.

Makes 3 cups, serving 8 to 18

NUTTY SPREAD

2 tablespoons walnut oil

4 ounces ground filbert nuts

1 tablespoon raw almond
butter (see Nut Butter recipe,
page 197)

⅛ teaspoon powdered raw
cayenne pepper

¼ teaspoon paprika

1 tablespoon dried garlic
powder

½ cup chopped olives

½ red bell pepper, minced

Blend all ingredients except the olives and red bell pepper until smooth. Stir in the olives and bell pepper. To enhance the flavor, allow to sit for several hours before serving. Spread on top of thinly sliced zucchini or yellow squash circles.

Makes 6 to 8 servings

SOFT SQUASH SENSATION

¼ cup pure extra virgin olive oil

1 teaspoon chopped coriander
leaf

1 teaspoon minced thyme

2 medium zucchini or
yellow squash

Mix oil and seasonings together and dip or spread on squash that has been cut into long sections. Dehydrate for 8 hours.

Makes 6 to 8 servings

RED PEPPER AND ONION ZIP

3 red or yellow bell peppers
2 large Vidalia onions

¼ small garlic clove
¼ cup ground sprouted rye

Blend all ingredients together on medium speed for 4 minutes. Roll mixture into balls about the size of golf balls and dehydrate for 12 hours.

Makes 6 to 8 servings

SEAFOOD TEMPTATIONS

4 ounces dried arame*
1 ounce dulse*
1 garlic clove

¼ cup ground spelt*
1 (25 gram) package nori*

Blend the arame, dulse, garlic, and spelt together on medium speed for 2 minutes.

   Spread about 4 ounces of the spelt mixture on a piece of nori and roll it up tightly. Cut into 3 to 5 pieces. Repeat the process until all of the spelt mixture is used.

Makes 4 to 6 servings

THE HOLY PROTEIN ROLLER

1 cup ground organic almonds
1 cup ground organic sunflower
   seeds

1 ounce powdered cloves
¼ cup pure water*

(continued)

Blend all the ingredients on medium speed for 1 minute. Let sit for 1 hour. Use as a dip for dried vegetables.

Makes 4 to 6 servings

GRAIN TASTY

1 cup ground kamut* sprouts
1 cup ground buckwheat
   sprouts
1 cup spelt sprouts
6 drops liquid stevia*

1 teaspoon cinnamon
⅛ cup pure water*
   Basic Pie Crust (see
   page 232)

Blend all ingredients on medium speed for 5 minutes. Pour mixture into pie crust. Chill pie for about 2 hours and cut into thin pie-shaped slices.

Makes 8 to 12 servings

BEAN KING DIP

2 cups sprouted Northern
   white beans
¼ cup pure water*

1 cup sprouted red beans
2 garlic cloves

Blend all the ingredients on medium speed for 5 minutes. Pour into a decorative bowl and place lettuce leaves around the sides. Use as a dip for dried vegetables.

Makes 6 to 8 servings

PICASSO SALSA

1 red bell pepper

1 yellow bell pepper

1 purple bell pepper

1 cup mung bean sprouts

½ teaspoon powdered raw cayenne pepper

Chop half of the peppers and sprouts finely and place in a decorative bowl. Blend the remaining ingredients on medium speed for 3 minutes. Pour mixture into bowl with chopped ingredients and stir well.

Makes 4 to 6 servings

Breads

Essene Rye Crisp

4 cups sprouted rye
½ cup pure water*

1 teaspoon caraway seeds
(optional)

Blend all ingredients for 3 minutes on high speed. Pour mixture into a solid dehydrator tray. Dehydrate for 8 to 10 hours.

Makes 3 to 4 servings

MULTI-GRAIN THIN BREAD

1 cup sprouted quinoa*
1 cup sprouted amaranth*
⅛ cup pure water*

1 cup buckwheat sprouts
1 cup millet sprouts

Blend all ingredients for 3 minutes on medium speed. Pour mixture into a solid dehydrator tray to desired thickness. Dehydrate for 24 hours.

Makes 3 to 4 servings

SPANISH CRACKER

4 cups spelt* sprouts
1 teaspoon powdered raw
   cayenne pepper

¼ cup pure water*

Blend all the ingredients together for 3 minutes on medium speed. Pour mixture into solid dehydrator tray. Dehydrate for 16 hours. If desired, break cracker into tortilla-chip-sized pieces.

Makes 3 to 4 servings

ITALIAN WHOLE BREAD

2 cups sprouted oats
2 cups sprouted kamut*
1 cup sprouted spelt*
⅛ cup pure water*

2 tablespoons extra virgin
   olive oil
1 teaspoon oregano

Blend all the ingredients together for 2 minutes on medium speed. Pour mixture into solid dehydrator tray to desired thickness. Dehydrate for 24 hours.

Makes 3 to 4 servings

Breads

TASTY GRAINY STUFF

½ cup sprouted barley
½ cup sprouted rye
½ cup sprouted millet
½ cup sprouted spelt*
½ cup sprouted kamut*

½ cup sprouted oats
½ cup pure water*
1 teaspoon cinnamon
1 teaspoon powdered
    stevia*

Blend all ingredients together for 4 minutes on medium speed. Pour mixture in small circles onto a solid dehydrator tray. If desired, place herbs on top of each grain circle. Dehydrate for 12 to 24 hours.

Makes 4 to 6 servings

SPROUTED GRAIN BREAD

8 to 12 cups of any sprouted
        grain (see Hippocrates
        Sprouting Chart, page 170)

Grind sprouted grain in a food processor or juicer. Form ground grain sprouts into a loaf. Dehydrate for 24 hours.

Makes 1 large loaf, or 2 to 3 medium loaves

Butter Substitute Spreads

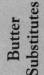

Nut Butter

2 cups shelled raw almonds
  or hulled raw sunflower seeds

Run nuts through a Champion-type juicer with the homogenization blank. If you do not have this type of juicer, finely grind the nuts without separating out the oil.

Store unused nut butter in a glass jar in the refrigerator for up to three days. (Do not eat with bread, however. Spread it on dehydrated vegetables.)

Makes 4 to 5 servings

SQUASH SPREAD

1 cup cubed Hubbard squash   ½ cup sprouted barley
½ cup cubed butternut squash   ¼ cup pure water*
1 tablespoon grapeseed oil

Blend all the ingredients for 1 to 2 minutes. Transfer to a container
and refrigerate for up to three days.
     Use on sprouted breads.

Makes 2 to 4 servings

SWEETSTUFF SPREAD

1 cup chopped sweet potatoes   1 teaspoon nutmeg
1 cup chopped yams   ¼ cup pure water*
2 teaspoons walnut oil

Blend all the ingredients for 1 to 2 minutes. Transfer to a container
and refrigerate for up to three days. Use on all types of whole grain
sprouted breads.

Makes 3 to 4 servings

Soups

These soups make delicious cold meals. But if you like, you can gently warm the soups to 110 degrees F. Heating to this level will not destroy the soups' natural enzyme, oxygen, and nutrient content.

BUTTERNUT SMOOTH SOUP

1 butternut squash, peeled, seeded, and sliced
1 yellow bell pepper
4 stalks celery
1 red onion
1 teaspoon curry

½ cup raw almond butter (see page 197)
½ teaspoon nutmeg
Braggs Aminos* to taste
¼ cup pure water*

Blend all ingredients and add enough pure water to create desired consistency. For decoration, float edible flowers on top.

Makes 2 to 4 servings

WINTER SOUP MEAL

3 cups sunflower greens
1 cup mung bean sprouts
1 ounce dulse*
1 cup sprouted greens
1 cup chopped watercress

½ cup sunflower seed meal*
¼ cup pure water*
2 to 4 tablespoons minced onion
¼ teaspoon powdered raw
    cayenne pepper

Combine the sunflower greens, mung bean sprouts, and dulse in a large bowl. Blend the remaining ingredients to a smooth consistency. Pour over the greens, sprouts, and dulse.

Variation: Substitute a mixture of comfrey and buckwheat greens, or lettuce and mustard greens for the sunflower greens. If using mustard greens, omit the cayenne pepper.

Makes 2 to 4 servings

VEGETABLE SOUP

1 red bell pepper
½ small cucumber
¼ cup sliced green beans
1 small onion, sliced
¼ sweet potato or yam
2 to 3 cabbage leaves

2 to 3 spinach or chard leaves
½ cup pure water*
1 teaspoon vegetable
    seasoning
¼ teaspoon dulse*

Blend all the ingredients until smooth and creamy. Any vegetables in season may be substituted.

Makes 4 to 6 servings

Basic Seed Soup

½ cup seeds (sunflower,
  almond, sesame, pumpkin,
  or sprouted chickpeas)
1 to 2 cups pure water*
  1 cup sprouts (any variety)
  1 cup grated squash
    (summer, zucchini, or
    Hubbard)

1 tablespoon minced onion
1 tablespoon minced garlic
¼ teaspoon powdered raw
  cayenne pepper

Grind the seeds to a fine powder and soak in 1 cup of the pure water for about 8 hours. Put in blender, add the sprouts, add enough pure water to achieve desired texture. Before serving, stir in the squash, onion, garlic, and cayenne pepper.

For more tang, blend additional onion and garlic into soup instead of stirring it in at the end. For a thicker texture, add more ground seed.

Makes 2 to 4 servings

Green Avocado Soup

1 large, ripe avocado
2 cups indoor salad greens
  (such as buckwheat or
  sunflower)
1 cup pure water*

2 tablespoons grapeseed oil
1 teaspoon chives
1 teaspoon kelp*
1 teaspoon tamari*

Blend all the ingredients until smooth. If you prefer a thicker soup, add ¼ cup sunflower seed meal or an extra avocado.

Makes 2 to 4 servings

CREAMY VEGETABLE SOUP

1 pound young and tender   ½ bunch watercress
  green beans   1 teaspoon kelp*
1 onion   Dash powdered raw
2 yellow squash   cayenne pepper (optional)
3 celery stalks   ¼ cup pure water*

Clean and mince the vegetables and watercress. Blend all the ingredients until creamy.

Makes 2 to 4 servings

KALE GREENS SOUP

2 cups kale greens (no stems)   1 carrot, julienned
2 garlic cloves, chopped   4 reiki mushrooms
1 cup snap peas   3 teaspoons Braggs Aminos*
2 green onions, chopped   ¼ cup pure water*

Blend all ingredients together until creamy.

Makes 2 to 4 servings

SPROUTED CORN PORRIDGE

2 cups dried organic corn   2 tablespoons pure water*

Sprout the corn for 2 days. Purée sprouted corn in a blender and serve.

Makes 2 servings

AUTUMN SOUP

1 cup young, tender brussels
  sprouts
1 large onion
2 garlic cloves
1 leek
½ cup cauliflower florets
¼ cup pure water*

½ peeled butternut squash
½ bunch parsley, chopped
2 stalks celery, chopped
½ head small red cabbage
3 kale stalks
⅛ cup vegetable seasoning

Blend all ingredients together until creamy.

Makes 4 servings

BARLEY SOUP

1 cup sprouted barley
1 garlic clove
½ pound mushrooms
1½ onions
1 parsnip
2 celery stalks
¼ head red cabbage, sliced
¼ cup pure water*

2 tablespoons grapeseed oil
1 teaspoon dried parsley
2 tablespoons minced basil
  Braggs Aminos* to taste
2 tablespoons organic
  herbal mix (found in
  health food stores)

Blend all ingredients together until creamy.

Makes 2 to 4 servings

KALE, CABBAGE, AND SPROUTED BEAN SOUP

3 cups chopped kale
2 cups minced cabbage
1 cup sprouted baby
   lima beans
1 strip kombu*, 6 inches
   long

1½ cups minced onion
1 teaspoon savory
¼ cup barley miso*
5 cups pure water*
¼ cup pure water*

Soak dried baby lima beans 8 hours or overnight and sprout for 2 days. Blend all ingredients together until creamy. If soup is too thick, add more water.

Makes 4 to 6 servings

RAW CELERY SOUP

½ cup fresh celery juice
½ cup fresh carrot juice
   Juice of ½ lemon
1 teaspoon almond meal*
1 teaspoon sesame seed meal*
3 teaspoons grapeseed oil

½ red bell pepper
2 to 4 tablespoon minced raw
   cayenne pepper
2 to 4 tablespoon minced onion
2 to 4 tablespoons minced celery
1 garlic clove, pressed

Blend the juices and the meals on medium speed until creamy. Add oil and blend again. Transfer to a large bowl. Stir in remaining ingredients.

Makes 2 servings

Salads

AVOCADO SALAD

2 ripe, but firm, avocados
1 cup snow peas, stemmed
2 tablespoons minced thyme
½ teaspoon radish sprouts

¼ teaspoon powdered raw
  cayenne pepper
Braggs Aminos* to taste

Peel and slice the avocados. Gently hand-mix the avocados with the remaining ingredients.

Makes 3 to 4 servings

LEAFY AVOCADO SALAD

2 ripe, but firm, avocados
½ bunch spinach
½ bunch watercress
1 head Bibb lettuce
1 bunch green onions,
   green part only

2 sprigs fresh mint, minced
4 red radishes, minced
Juice of 1 lemon
Braggs Aminos* to taste

Cut avocados in half, remove the pits and scoop into balls with a melon baller. Clean and chop the greens. Mince the green onions. Combine all the ingredients together, tossing with the lemon juice and Braggs Aminos.

Makes 3 to 4 servings

ALMOST TUNA SALAD

1 red bell pepper
½ cup chopped celery
2 to 3 tablespoons seed sauce*
2 to 3 tablespoons raw almond
   butter (see Nut Butter
   recipe, page 197)

1 tablespoon kelp*
   (or more to taste)
¼ cup mung bean sprouts
¼ cup lentil sprouts
¼ cup chopped onion
¼ cup chopped parsley
1 cup alfalfa sprouts

Cut the red pepper in half and scrape out the ribs and seeds. Set aside.
   Blend the celery, seed sauce, almond butter, and kelp on medium speed until smooth. Add the mung bean sprouts, lentil sprouts, onion, and ⅛ cup of the parsley. Pulse blender for a few seconds until the sprouts are slightly chopped. Stir the blended mixture into the alfalfa sprouts. Serve in the red pepper cups and garnish with the remaining parsley.

Makes 2 to 4 servings

CAULIFLOWER SALAD
WITH SUNFLOWER SAUCE

Salad
½ head cauliflower, cut into
   bite-size pieces
3 red bell peppers, chopped
½ yellow bell pepper, chopped
½ cup parsley, minced
1 tablespoon marjoram

Sauce
1 cup coarsely ground
   sunflower seed sprouts
1 cup pure water*
½ cup grated carrots

Combine the salad ingredients in a decorative serving bowl.

To make the sauce, purée the sunflower sprouts and pure water until smooth. Add the carrots and blend again. Pour the sauce over the vegetables before serving. Serve with indoor greens and mixed sprouts.

Variation: Substitute broccoli for the cauliflower.

Makes 4 to 6 servings

STUFFED PEPPERS

2 large bell peppers
1 cup wheat sprouts
¼ red pepper, minced
2 to 3 green beans, chopped

¼ cup fresh peas from pod
4 tablespoons grapeseed oil
1 tablespoon kelp*

Cut the tops off the peppers and scrape out the ribs and seeds. Combine remaining ingredients and stuff the peppers with the mixture.

Makes 2 servings

TOSSED GREEN SALAD

2 cups mixed romaine,
    endive, chicory, and/or
    other lettuces
¼ cup parsley, minced
¼ cup chives, minced

¼ cup watercress leaves
¼ cup minced green onions
    Juice of ½ lemon
2 tablespoons grapeseed oil
1 tablespoon almond meal*

Tear the greens into bite-size pieces. Mix with the parsley, chives, watercress, and green onions.

Mix the lemon juice and oil in a small jar. Shake well and pour over the greens. Toss well to coat. Sprinkle with the almond meal.

Makes 2 servings

HIPPOCRATES LUNCHEON SALAD

2 cups alfalfa sprouts
2 cups buckwheat lettuce
1 cup mung bean sprouts
½ cup fenugreek sprouts
½ cup sunflower seed sprouts
½ cup chopped zucchini

1 red bell pepper, chopped
1 tablespoon dulse*
    Basic Nut Sauce or
    Autumn Nut Sauce
    (see page 219)

Place all the ingredients in a large salad bowl and serve with nut sauce of choice.

Makes 4 servings

DANDELION SALAD

1 cup alfalfa sprouts
10 to 12 dandelion leaves,
    torn into bite-size pieces

1 red bell pepper, sliced
1 leek, white part only,
    sliced

Place alfalfa sprouts on a serving platter. Top with remaining ingredients.

Makes 4 servings

CARROT-RUTABAGA SALAD

6 large carrots, grated
1 large rutabaga, grated
2 tablespoons flaxseed oil
2 tablespoons lime juice

3 tablespoons dried oregano,
    or 6 tablespoons fresh
Braggs Aminos* to taste

Combine all the ingredients. Refrigerate for 1 hour before serving.

Makes 3 to 4 servings

BROCCOLI AND CAULIFLOWER SALAD

⅓ cup canola oil
1 tablespoon Braggs Aminos*
1 teaspoon prepared
    horseradish
1 teaspoon ground mustard
½ teaspoon tarragon

¼ cup minced onion
4 cups bite-size broccoli
    florets
2 cups bite-size cauliflower
    florets

(continued)

Combine the oil, Braggs Aminos, horseradish, mustard, tarragon, and onion. Let stand for 10 minutes, then pour over the broccoli and cauliflower. Toss lightly and refrigerate for 30 minutes before serving. (Lightly toss the salad a few times while it is being chilled.)

Makes 4 servings

CORN AND MUSHROOM SALAD

4 ears corn
1 pound fresh shiitake
   mushrooms, sliced
3 to 4 garlic cloves, chopped
   finely
2 cups radish sprouts
1 teaspoon fennel seeds

½ teaspoon powdered raw
   cayenne pepper
Juice of 2 limes
Braggs Aminos* to taste
Red bell pepper and
   paprika for garnish

Cut the corn kernels off the cob. Mix all the ingredients well. Garnish with diced red pepper and paprika.

Makes 2 to 4 servings

ORANGE AND SUN SALAD

6 cups coarsely shredded
   carrot
8 ounces green olives, halved

½ cup chopped basil
2 tablespoons lime juice

Mix all ingredients and serve.

Makes 2 to 4 servings

RAW COLESLAW

4 ounces raw tahini*
1 garlic clove
   Pure water* as needed
2 cups shredded red cabbage
2 cups shredded
   green cabbage
2 tablespoons juniper
   berries

2 tablespoons dill seeds,
   crushed
2 tablespoons caraway
   seeds, crushed
   Braggs Aminos* to taste

Blend the tahini and garlic. Add enough pure water until desired thickness is achieved. Pour sauce over cabbage, berries, and crushed seeds, and toss lightly. Season to taste with Braggs Aminos.

Makes 4 to 6 servings

POTATO AND SQUASH SALAD

3 cups cubed yellow squash
3 cups cubed zucchini
1 cup grated sweet potato
1 cup grated carrot
4 tablespoons finely
   chopped tarragon

3 garlic cloves, crushed
3 tablespoons cold-pressed
   olive or grapeseed oil
   Braggs Aminos* to taste

Combine all the ingredients in a bowl.

Makes 4 servings

SESAME BROCCOLI SALAD

Vegetables
2 cups broccoli florets
2 cups mung bean sprouts
1 cup sliced red bell pepper

Sauce
2 tablespoons sesame
  seed oil

2 tablespoons Braggs
  Aminos*
1 tablespoon chopped
  coriander leaf
½ teaspoon powdered raw
  cayenne pepper
¼ cup sesame seeds, soaked
  2 to 3 hours

Combine vegetables and place in a bowl. Purée the sauce ingredients and pour over the vegetables. Toss gently and let sit for 30 minutes before serving.

Makes 6 servings

COMPLETE MEAL SALAD

2 cups chopped sunflower
  greens
2 cups chopped buckwheat
  lettuce
2 cups clover sprouts

1 cup lentil or mung
  bean sprouts
1 to 2 celery stalks, chopped
3 red bell peppers,
  chopped

Toss all the ingredients together. Serve with your favorite homemade dressing (see "Dressings" recipes).

Makes 4 servings

SALAD ROLLS

1 avocado
2 cups clover sprouts
1 cup mung bean sprouts
1 large red bell pepper

1 dash Braggs Aminos*
10 outer leaves romaine
   lettuce, or 4 sheets nori*

Mash the avocado with a fork. Add the sprouts, red pepper, and Braggs Aminos and mix well. Place a portion of the mixture on each lettuce leaf or nori sheet. Roll up into cylinders.

Makes 2 to 4 servings

SIMPLE BROCCOLI

2 cups broccoli, cut into
   bite-size pieces
2 cups cauliflower, cut into
   bite-size pieces
1 cup sprouted whole
   almonds

Raw almond butter (see Nut
   Butter recipe, page 197)
   blended with water for
   taste

Mix all ingredients together and serve.

Makes 2 to 4 servings

Dressings

CUCUMBER DILL DRESSING

1 large cucumber
5 ounces uncooked tempeh*
1 onion
1 garlic clove
1 tablespoon raw tahini*

3 tablespoon dried dill
4 ounces plain rice milk
Organic vegetable flakes
to taste
1 tablespoon pure water*

Peel and seed the cucumber. Place all the ingredients in a blender and liquefy.

Variations: Substitute 1 tablespoon basil or ¾ teaspoon cumin for the dill. If you want more zip, add a pinch or two of powdered raw cayenne pepper.

Makes 3 to 5 servings

SQUASH AVOCADO DRESSING

2 ripe avocados, peeled
  and pitted
2 zucchini, peeled and
  chopped
3 chopped green onions

1 garlic clove
½ cup chopped thyme
  Braggs Aminos* to taste
2 tablespoons pure water*

Blend all the ingredients together, reserving a handful of chopped green onion for garnish, and add enough pure water until desired consistency is reached. Garnish with green onions and chill.

Variations: Substitute cilantro, dill, or oregano for the thyme.

Makes 2 to 4 servings

GREEN GODDESS DRESSING

¼ cup ground hazelnuts
½ cup chopped basil
2 garlic cloves
1 chopped onion
1 cup buckwheat sprouts
1 cup shredded green
  cabbage

1 cup sunflower spouts
2 tablespoons fresh ginger
  juice
2 green onions, minced,
  for garnish
¼ cup pure water*

Blend all the ingredients, adding enough pure water to reach desired consistency. Garnish with the green onions.

Makes 3 to 5 servings

Olive Basil Dressing

½ cup raw almond butter
  (see Nut Butter recipe,
  page 197)
½ cup pitted cured olives
½ cup dill

1 tablespoon basil
¼ teaspoon thyme
1 onion, chopped
  Braggs Aminos* to taste
2 tablespoons pure water*

Blend all the ingredients, adding enough pure water desired consistency is reached.

Makes 2 to 4 servings

A Touch of Italy Dressing

1 cucumber, peeled and
  minced
3 garlic cloves
1 tablespoon Italian
  seasoning

3 celery stalks, sliced
2 red bell peppers,
  chopped
2 tablespoons pure water*
  Parsley for garnish

Blend all ingredients together, adding enough pure water to reach desired consistency. Garnish with parsley and chill for about 1 hour.

Makes 3 to 5 servings

Tahini Dressing

3 garlic cloves
8 ounces raw tahini*

Braggs Aminos* to taste
2 tablespoons pure water*

(continued)

Blend all ingredients together, adding enough pure water until dressing is smooth and liquefied.

Variations: This basic recipe can be spiced up with many additional ingredients. Try onions, green onions, leeks, shallots, nutmeg, cinnamon, or dried red pepper.

Makes 2 to 4 servings

GREEN DRESSING

1 large avocado
1 small onion, quartered
2 celery stalks, cut into
  2-inch pieces
¼ cup parsley
¼ cup dill

¼ cup basil
¼ cup watercress
1 cucumber, unpeeled and
  quartered
1 garlic clove
  Braggs Aminos* to taste

Blend all ingredients in a blender, adding enough cucumber juice to reach desired thickness.

Makes 3 to 5 servings

SUNFLOWER-SWEET PEPPER DRESSING

1 cup sunflower seeds,
  soaked 3 to 5 hours
2 to 3 garlic cloves
½ cup chopped basil

2 tablespoons pure water*
2 to 3 cups red bell pepper
  chunks

Blend the sunflower seeds, garlic, and basil with enough pure water until creamy. Slowly add the red pepper and blend until smooth.

Makes 2 to 4 servings

PECAN DELIGHT DRESSING

2 cups pecans, soaked for   ½ cup coarsely chopped
   12 hours   parsley
2 to 3 garlic cloves   Braggs Aminos* to taste
   ¼ cup diced red onion   Cucumber juice

Blend all ingredients together, adding enough cucumber juice until creamy.

Makes 2 to 4 servings

SPINACH DRESSING

1 avocado   ½ bunch watercress
½ cup pure water*   ⅛ teaspoon fresh ginger
1 cup spinach leaves   ⅛ teaspoon kelp*
2 tablespoons pure water*

Blend the avocado with the pure water until creamy. Add in remaining ingredients and blend until smooth.

Makes 3 to 5 servings

LEMON HEALTH-ONNAISE DRESSING

Juice of ½ lemon   2 ounces agar flakes*
⅛ cup walnut oil   1 tablespoon pure water*

Combine all ingredients in a blender and liquefy to desired thickness.

Makes 2 to 4 servings

AVOCADO-SWEET PEPPER DRESSING

1 avocado, peeled and pitted
½ teaspoon dried coriander
  leaf

¼ cup pure water*
1 red, yellow, or pink bell
  pepper, finely chopped

Blend the avocado and coriander in the pure water on medium speed for 30 seconds. Add bell pepper, reserving a handful, and blend again. Stir in reserved bell pepper.

Makes 3 to 5 servings

BASIC NUT SAUCE

½ to 1 cup sprouted almond,
    hazelnut, and/or pine nuts
3 to 4 ounces pure water* for
    each ½ cup sprouts
1 garlic clove
2 tablespoons pure water*

1 green onion
⅛ teaspoon powdered raw
    cayenne pepper
1 leaf basil, oregano, or
    thyme

Blend all ingredients until puréed.

Makes 2 to 4 servings

AUTUMN NUT SAUCE

1 cup walnuts or pecans
4 ounces pure water*
½ medium leek

1 medium bunch
    peppermint or spearmint
2 tablespoons pure water*

Blend all ingredients on medium speed until puréed.

Makes 2 to 4 servings

Main Courses

LENTIL LOAF

1 cup sesame-sunflower
    seed meal*
A few tablespoons pure
    water*
2 cups sprouted red lentils

1 to 2 carrots, shredded
½ to 1 cup chopped celery
½ to 1 cup chopped red bell
    pepper
¼ cup pure water*

Mix the seed meal with the pure water to form a doughlike consistency and set aside.

Chop the lentils in a blender. Add the carrots, celery, and red pepper and blend on medium speed until creamy. Mix the lentil mixture with the seed meal mixture. Shape into a loaf. Serve.

Makes 6 servings

Asparagus with Shakti Mushrooms

Asparagus Mixture
1 pound asparagus
2 tablespoons grapeseed oil
½ cup finely chopped onions
2 cups sliced shakti
   mushrooms

Sauce
¼ cup pure water*
1 tablespoon lime juice
1 tablespoon Braggs
   Aminos* to taste
1½ teaspoons arrowroot

Combine the asparagus, grapeseed oil, onions, and mushrooms in a bowl. Blend the sauce ingredients for 1 minute and pour over the asparagus mixture.

Makes 4 servings

Rose Sauerkraut

4 heads red cabbage
2 apples, cored and cut
   into quarters

3 strips wakame*

Remove the outer leaves from the cabbages, rinse, and set aside. Finely chop 2 of the heads and set aside. Cut the other 2 heads into small pieces, place in blender, and blend until chunky. Mix the blended cabbage with the finely chopped cabbage and place in a container or crock. Place the apples on top of the cabbage and push down. Cover with the wakame. Line the inside of the exposed container walls with the reserved cabbage leaves.

   Clean the sides of the crock to keep from spoiling. Fill a plastic bag with water and close tightly, placing it on top of contents to seal

(continued)

the crock. Cover with a towel and ferment for 3 to 5 days in a cool, dark place. After fermenting throw away the top layer of cabbage leaves. Remove the wakame and serve as a side dish. Remove the apples and discard. Transfer the sauerkraut to another container and refrigerate for up to 2 months.

Makes 16 to 24 servings

PINE NUT PATTY

3 cups pine nuts
1/2 cup chopped red onion
1/2 cup chopped celery
1 package (4 ounces) agar flakes*

1½ cup chopped red bell pepper
Braggs Aminos* to taste
2 tablespoons pure water*

Combine all ingredients. Form into patties and serve.

Makes 4 servings

SESAME SENSATION

1 carrot, sliced
4 green onions, sliced
2 celery stalks, sliced
1 cup hulled sesame seeds
1 cup raw tahini*
2 teaspoons lemon juice

½ teaspoon dried dill
1 teaspoon dried basil
¼ cup chopped parsley
½ cup raw sauerkraut
Braggs Aminos* to taste
¼ cup pure water*

Blend all ingredients into a creamy paté. Mold and serve with fresh vegetables.

Makes 6 servings

HOMEY HUMMUS

1 large sweet potato
3 cups sprouted chickpeas
2 large garlic cloves
1 teaspoon oregano
½ teaspoon powdered raw
   cayenne pepper

1 teaspoon paprika
Braggs Aminos* to taste
Pure water*

Blend all the ingredients, adding enough pure water, if necessary, to make a thick paste. Serve with vegetables.

Makes 6 servings

CAULIFLOWER CURRY

2 tablespoons grapeseed oil
1 teaspoon minced ginger
½ to 1 teaspoon cumin
½ teaspoon tumeric
1 large onion, chopped

1 head cauliflower, cut into
   bite-size florets
¼ cup pure water*
½ teaspoon Braggs Aminos*
⅓ cup whole raw almonds

Mix all ingredients together and serve. Decorate with edible flowers.

Makes 6 servings

Sprouted Quinoa with Green Onions and Reiki Mushrooms

½ cup sprouted quinoa
3 medium green onions,
   chopped
1 tablespoon walnut oil

1 teaspoon tarragon
1 cup sliced reiki
   mushrooms
1 cup hot pure water*

Mix all ingredients together. Let sit for 10 minutes before serving.

Makes 4 servings

Rutabaga and Sweet Potato Dream

1 medium rutabaga,
   chopped finely
1 large or 2 small sweet
   potatoes, chopped finely

1 teaspoon tarragon
1 cup hot pure water*
4 tablespoons Braggs
   Aminos*

Combine all ingredients. Let sit for 20 minutes before serving.

Makes 4 servings

Cauliflower Loaf

1 cup shelled dried almonds,
   soaked for 6 hours in
   2 cups pure water*
1½ cups grated cauliflower
4 to 5 reiki mushrooms, grated
½ celery stalk, chopped

¼ green onion, diced
1 garlic clove, pressed
½ teaspoon dried basil
½ teaspoon dried ground
   sage

(continued)

Grind almonds as finely as possible. Mix all ingredients well and shape into a loaf. Serve on a bed of lettuce with salad or soup.

Makes 6 servings

SPROUT LOAF

1 cup alfalfa sprouts
1 cup lentil sprouts
1 cup mung bean sprouts
½ cup cabbage sprouts
1 cup shelled raw almonds, ground

1 celery stalk, diced
1 green onion, diced
½ red bell pepper, diced
  Braggs Aminos* to taste
  Pure water*

Mix ingredients in a bowl, adding just enough pure water to allow mixture to hold shape. Form mixture into a loaf. Serve on a bed of romaine lettuce.

Makes 6 servings

GUACAMOLE DINNER

2 to 4 avocados, peeled and pitted
1 red bell pepper, chopped
1 green onion, chopped
1 garlic clove, pressed

¼ cup mustard or onion sprouts (optional)
¼ teaspoon powedered raw cayenne pepper

Mash the avocados and mix with the other ingredients. Serve with salad.

Makes 4 to 8 servings

FILLED PEPPERS

3 cups chickpea sprouts
½ cup raw tahini*
1 celery stalk, diced
¼ cup finely chopped
   parsley
1 garlic clove, chopped

¼ teaspoon thyme
   Braggs Aminos* to taste
6 red bell peppers, topped
   and cleaned
¼ cup pure water*

Blend all ingredients except the peppers into a smooth, thick paste, sometimes shutting off the blender and hand stirring. Stuff mixture into peppers.

Makes 6 to 8 servings

WHEAT CASSEROLE

2 cups wheat sprouts
¼ cup sesame seeds sprouts
1 cup sunflower seed sprouts
1 cup raw walnuts
1 zucchini, shredded

1 celery stalk, diced
1 teaspoon dried ground
   sage
1 teaspoon Braggs Aminos*
2 tablespoons pure water*

Chop the sprouts and walnuts in a blender to a coarse consistency. Transfer to a bowl. Add the zucchini, celery, sage, and Braggs Aminos and mix well. Shape on a casserole dish and serve.

Makes 6 servings

KASHA PILAF

2½ cups pure water*
2 tablespoons Braggs Aminos*
2 cups sprouted buckwheat kasha
½ cup diced celery
½ cup fresh peas

½ cup diced carrots
½ cup diced onion
½ cup diced zucchini
Chopped watercress for garnish

Heat the water to 110 degrees F. Add the Braggs Aminos and kasha. Add the vegetables and allow them to absorb the liquid. Fluff with a fork. Garnish with the watercress.

Makes 4 servings

HUMMUS WITH SPELT PITAS

4 cups chickpeas
½ cup raw tahini*
6 to 8 large garlic cloves
Pure water*
Lemon juice to taste

Braggs Aminos* to taste
Powdered raw cayenne pepper to taste
6 spelt pitas (available at health food stores)

Blend the chickpeas until smooth. Add the tahini and garlic and blend until smooth. Add enough pure water as needed to reach a smooth, creamy consistency. Season with lemon juice, Braggs Aminos* and cayenne to taste. Serve with spelt pitas, sprouts and grated cucumbers and/or grated vegetables. Store leftovers in the refrigerator in a well-sealed container.

Makes 6 servings

LENTIL PIE

2 medium red bell peppers
2 tablespoons pure water*
1½ cups sprouted lentils
3 cups hot pure water*
1 tablespoon raw sesame oil
1 stalk celery, chopped
1 medium onion, chopped

1 teaspoon thyme
1 teaspoon cinnamon
¼ teaspoon cloves, finely chopped
¼ cup tamari*
1 Basic Pie Crust (see page 232)

Purée the red peppers with the pure water to make a paste. Mix in all the remaining ingredients. Pour into pie shell and let sit for 1 hour before serving.

Makes 6 servings

LENTIL LOAF

1 cup sesame-sunflower seed meal*
Pure water*
2 cups sprouted red lentils

1 to 2 carrots, well shredded
½ cup chopped red bell pepper
½ cup chopped fennel

Mix the seed meal with a few tablespoons of pure water to form a doughlike consistency. Set aside.

Chop the lentils in the blender. Add the vegetables and blend on medium speed until creamy. Transfer mixture to a bowl. Add the seed meal mixture and mix all together. Shape into a loaf.

Makes 4 servings

BUCKWHEAT GREEN STEM PASTA

½ cup Italian parsley
2 garlic cloves
3 cups basil
2 tablespoons pure water*

¼ cup walnut oil
16 cups buckwheat green
stems (see note)

Blend the parsley, garlic, basil, water, and oil to a saucelike consistency. Pour over the stem "pasta."

Makes 4 to 6 servings

Note: To obtain green stems, cut the flowers off of buckwheat green sprouts and reserve the long stems.

VEGETABLE SEED LOAF

1 cup sunflower seed meal*
1 cup almond meal*
1 cup sesame seed meal*
½ cup pure water*
4 to 5 diced reiki mushrooms
½ cup diced parsley

3 stalks celery, diced
2 garlic cloves, diced
1 tablespoon Braggs
Aminos*
1 teaspoon basil

Mix all ingredients well. Shape into a loaf and chill overnight.

Makes 6 servings

Spicy Chickpea Sprouts

3 cups sprouted chickpeas
4 to 6 tablespoons grapeseed oil
¼ cup parsley, minced

¼ cup minced onion
1 tablespoon paprika
1 teaspoon herbal mix

Mash the chickpeas in the oil, using a potato masher, mortar and pestle, or blender. Add to remaining ingredients and mix well.

Makes 4 servings

Sunflower Rollups

1 red bell pepper
2½ cups day-old sunflower
    seed sprouts
1 teaspoon Braggs Aminos*,
    kelp*, or dulse*
2 tablespoons pure water*

1 cup alfalfa sprouts
1 small zucchini or yellow
    squash, diced
¼ cup diced celery
¼ cup diced green onion
6 sheets nori*

Blend red pepper until thoroughly liquefied. Add the sunflower sprouts, lemon juice, and Braggs Aminos* and blend on medium speed until smooth. Transfer mixture to a bowl. Add remaining ingredients, except for nori, and mix well. Place a portion of the sunflower mixture on each piece of nori and roll up into a cylinder. Pat the edges of the nori with a little water to seal. Place rollups on a serving plate surrounded by baby salad greens.

Makes 6 to 12 servings

WHEAT CASSEROLE

2 cups wheat sprouts
¼ cup dry unhulled sesame
   seeds, soaked 6 hours in
   ½ cup pure water*
1 cup sunflower sprouts
1 cup shelled raw walnuts,
   soaked 6 hours in 2 cups
   pure water*

1 zucchini, shredded
1 celery stalk, diced
1 teaspoon ground parsley
1 teaspoon Braggs Aminos*
2 tablespoons pure water*

Blend the wheat sprouts, sesame seeds, sunflower sprouts, and walnuts until mealy. Transfer to a bowl. Add the remaining ingredients and mix well. Mold into a casserole dish.

Makes 6 servings

Desserts

Please note that some of the following recipes are not perfect food combinations.

BASIC PIE CRUST

1 cup raw almonds	1 teaspoon cinnamon
½ cup mixture of dates, figs, and raisins	1 tablespoon pure water*

Chop the almonds in a blender until coarse. Add the remaining ingredients and blend again. Press mixture into a 10-inch pie pan.

Makes 1 crust

YAM PIE

1 cup pitted dates
2 cups walnuts
1 Basic Pie Crust (see page 232)
6 medium yams or sweet
  potatoes
½ cup sunflower seeds
2 tablespoons pure water*

½ teaspoon five-spice
  powder
2 tablespoons psyllium
  powder*
1 teaspoon coriander leaf
  Pine nuts for garnish

Blend ½ cup of the dates with the walnuts and a couple teaspoons of water in a blender. Press date mixture into the pie crust and set aside.

Peel and slice the yams; purée them in a juicer alternating with the nuts and dates. Add remaining ingredients and mix well. Press into pie crust. Garnish with pine nuts and chill.

Makes 1 pie

FRESH ORGANIC FRUIT PIE

3 cups sliced fruit (any kind)
1 Basic Pie Crust (see page 232)
1 cup apple juice
1 tablespoon agar powder*
  dissolved in ¼ cup
  pure water*

3 tablespoons agar flakes*
½ teaspoon cinnamon
1 teaspoon nonalcoholic
  vanilla

Place the fruit into the pie crust. Heat the apple juice with the agar flakes at 110 degrees F. for 15 minutes; stir in the vanilla and cinnamon. Pour apple juice mixture over fruit and chill until firm.

Makes 1 pie

MINCEY PIE

¼ cup currants
½ cup dried unsweetened
  papaya
½ cup raisins
½ cup dried figs (no stems)
  Pure water*
1 pear, cored
1 apple, cored
1 tablespoon lemon juice

1 tablespoon pumpkin pie
  spice
¼ teaspoon ground cloves
⅛ teaspoon nutmeg
2 tablespoons flax seeds,
  ground
1 Basic Pie Crust
  (see page 232)

Soak the currants, papaya, raisins, and figs in pure water* for several hours to soften; drain.

Chop the pear and apple and put into a blender with the soaked and drained fruit. Add the lemon juice, spices, and flax and blend on medium speed for 1 minute. Press into pie crust. Chill.

Makes 1 pie

NO-BAKE PUMPKIN PIE

3 cups blended pumpkin
3 tablespoons agar flakes*
½ teaspoon cinnamon
½ teaspoon mace
¼ teaspoon ground cloves

½ cup sweet potato purée
½ cup Hubbard squash
  purée
1 Basic Pie Crust (see
  page 232)

Place the pumpkin, agar flakes, and spices in a saucepan and heat to 110 degrees F., stirring until flakes are dissolved. Put pumpkin mixture into a blender and blend until smooth. Add the spices, sweet potatoes, and squash and mix. Pour into pie crust and chill for at least two hours.

Makes 1 pie

Avocado Cups

1 ripe avocado, peeled and
  pitted
4 apples, cored and chopped

2 tablespoons lemon juice
¼ cup pure water*

Blend all ingredients until smooth. Pour into glass custard cups and serve immediately.

Makes 4 servings

Old World Carrot Cake

1 cup black mission figs,
  soaked for 1 hour in
  ½ cup pure water*
⅔ cup raisins, soaked for
  1 hour in ½ cup
  pure water*
⅓ cup pitted dates, soaked
  for 1 hour in ½ cup
  pure water*

⅔ cup pine nuts
1 cup walnut pieces
4 cups finely grated carrot
1 cup shredded coconut
1 teaspoon ground
  cinnamon
½ teaspoon ground ginger
½ teaspoon ground cloves

Drain the fruit and put through a juicer. Place in a large bowl and knead in the remaining ingredients until well mixed. Mold into desired shape on a large serving plate. Decorate with nuts or edible flowers.

Makes 12 servings

CREAMY APPLE-WALNUT PUDDING

1 apple, peeled, cored, and
finely chopped
2 cups dried apples, soaked
for 6 hours or overnight
in 4 cups pure water*

1 cup shelled raw walnuts,
soaked for 6 hours or overnight in 2 cups pure water*
4 drops liquid stevia*
Cinnamon to taste

Reserve water from soaking apples and blend with the fruit and walnuts until creamy. Blend in stevia and cinnamon to taste.

Makes 6 servings

FLAMING FRUIT

2 cups ground almond meal
1 cup finely ground
hazelnuts
½ cup pure water*

1 mango, chopped
1 papaya, chopped
1 orange, chopped
1 tangerine, chopped

Blend the almond and hazelnuts with the pure water on medium speed until creamy. Place mixture in bottom of a pie pan. Toss the fruits together and place on top of the nut mixture.

Makes 6 servings

CAROB BANANA ICE-BARS

10 tablespoons raw carob
powder
5 to 10 tablespoons pure water*

4 firm bananas, peeled
4 Popsicle sticks

(continued)

Mix the carob powder with the water and warm to 110 degrees F., stirring mixture, until dissolved. Place an ice-bar stick into each banana and dip into the carob mixture. Wrap each dipped banana in a piece of waxed paper and place in freezer overnight, or until frozen.

Makes 4 servings

CAROB PUDDING

1 Hawaiian papaya, peeled and seeded	1 cup fresh carrot juice 2 tablespoons carob powder

Blend all ingredients together on medium speed. Pour mixture into 2 or 3 small custard dishes. Let sit in the refrigerator for 2 hours before serving.

Makes 2 to 3 servings

ALMOND BARS

¼ cup maple syrup 2 tablespoons arrowroot powder	2 cups soaked and sprouted almonds

Mix the maple syrup and arrowroot powder until thick. Place sprouted almonds in a blender and chop into tiny pieces. Add almonds to maple syrup mixture and form into bars on parchment paper. Place in the freezer for at least 1 hour before serving.

Makes 6 to 8 bars

Coconut-Banana Cream Pie

4 tablespoons agar flakes*
¼ cup pure water*
3 cups shredded coconut

8 pitted Majool dates,
   chopped
6 frozen bananas

Dissolve the agar in the water. Combine agar mixture with the coconut and dates; mix thoroughly. Place the mixture in a glass pie plate, forming a crust. Place in refrigerator and chill for 1 hour.

Blend the bananas until creamy. Pour into the pie crust and serve.

Makes 1 pie

Fudge

4 cups sprouted spelt*
5 tablespoons carob powder

5 drops liquid stevia*
2 tablespoons pure water*

Dehydrate the sprouted spelt for 24 hours, then grind into flour. Add the carob powder and stevia, and water and mix well. Spread mixture into a shallow pan.

Makes 6 servings

Juices and Drinks

All of the following juices are made by combining a variety of juices.
The measurement given for a juice is the amount after the ingredient
has been liquefied in a juicer. Because the amount of liquid in a fruit or
vegetable varies from one piece to the next, it's impossible to say
exactly how much is needed to produce the given measurement. Use
as much of the ingredient necessary to make the required quantity of
juice. Also remember: You should drinks these juices immediately after
juicing to maintain their nutrients, oxygen, and enzymes.

(Information on juicers can be found in chapter 9.)

FRUIT JUICE

4 ounces fruit juice (any kind)   8 ounces pure water*

(continued)

Combine ingredients and stir.

Note: An exaggerated amount of fructose (sugar) is found in fruit today due to hybridization. Fruit juices should be used sparingly and always diluted.

Makes 1 serving

LIVE VERT JUICE

1 ounce spearmint or
  peppermint juice
3 ounces anise juice

4 ounces celery juice
4 ounces parsnip juice

Combine all ingredients and stir well.

Makes 1 serving

GREEN JUICE HIPPOCRATES-STYLE

4 ounces sunflower green
  sprout juice
2 ounces buckwheat green
  sprout juice

6 ounces cucumber juice
6 ounces celery juice

Combine all ingredients.

Makes 1 serving

PUREST GREEN DRINK

7½ ounces sunflower green
    sprout juice
3½ ounces buckwheat green
    sprout juice

4 ounces clover sprout
  juice

Combine all ingredients.

Makes 1 serving

POWER PURE JUICE

4 ounces mixed baby
  greens juice
1 ounce thyme juice
1 ounce oregano juice

⅛ ounce garlic juice
10 ounces romaine lettuce
  juice

Combine all ingredients.

Makes 1 serving

HERBS IN A GLASS

1 ounce marjoram juice
1 ounce coriander juice
1 ounce thyme juice

1 ounce wintergreen juice
12 ounces cucumber juice

Combine all ingredients.

Makes 1 serving

A WILD, EDIBLE WEED DRINK

2 ounce lamb's-quarter
greens juice

2 ounces wild Queen Anne's
lace juice

2 ounces mint juice

5 ounces fennel juice

5 ounces celery juice

Combine all ingredients.

Note: Lamb's quarter and Queen Anne's lace may be found in your
yard or a nearby forest.

Makes 1 serving

GIVING LIQUID

5 ounces mung bean sprout
juice

2 ounces adzuki juice*

9 ounces winter squash
juice

Combine all ingredients.

Makes 1 serving

LIVING AND LOVING JUICE

2 ounces beet juice

2 ounces carrot juice

2 ounces celery juice

2 ounces cucumber juice

1 ounce parsley juice

1 ounce watercress juice

6 ounces iceberg lettuce
juice

Combine all ingredients.

Makes 1 serving

STANDARD HEALTH FOOD STORE JUICE

4 ounces carrot juice

4 ounces celery juice

2 ounces beet juice

6 ounces cucumber juice

Combine all ingredients.

Makes 1 serving

QUEEN'S JUICE

4 ounces jicama juice*

4 ounces sweet potato juice

4 ounces Hubbard squash juice

3 ounces yam juice

1 ounce mint juice

Combine all ingredients.

Makes 1 serving

WATERMELON COMPLETE

16 ounces whole watermelon, juiced (include rind, seeds, and red fruit)

This is an excellent kidney and bladder cleanser. But people with sugar sensitivity should avoid this drink.

Makes 1 serving

GRAPE-APPLE JUICE

8 ounces apple juice

8 ounces grape juice

Combine all ingredients.

Makes 1 serving

MELLOW MIX

4 ounces cantaloupe juice
(fruit only)

4 ounces honeydew melon
juice (fruit only)

4 ounces watermelon juice
(fruit and rind)

Combine all ingredients.

Makes 1 serving

SUMMER PASSION

4 ounces peach juice

4 ounces pear juice

4 ounces apple juice

Combine all ingredients.

Makes 1 serving

ITALIAN STALLION

8 ounces zucchini juice
7 ounces yellow summer
  squash juice

1 ounce garlic juice

Combine all ingredients.

Makes 1 serving

BASIC GREEN DRINK

4 ounces buckwheat green
  juice
4 ounces sunflower green
  juice

4 ounces alfalfa sprout juice
1 carrot, juiced
1 green onion, juiced
2 tablespoons sauerkraut

Combine all ingredients.

Makes 1 serving

RED-BLOODED AMERICAN

3 ounces alfalfa sprout juice
3 ounces mung bean sprout
  juice
3 ounces lentil sprout juice
1 kale leaf, juiced

3 ounces Jerusalem
  artichoke juice
1 ounce green beans, juiced
1 medium parsnip, juiced
1 ounce fennel juice

Combine all ingredients.

Makes 1 serving

WILD ONE

4 ounces sunflower green
   juice
2 ounces radish sprout juice
4 ounces buckwheat green
   juice

8 ounces lamb's-quarter juice
1 stalk celery, juiced
½ small zucchini, juiced
½ red bell pepper, juiced
½ beet, juiced

Combine all ingredients.

Makes 1 serving

SPRINGTIME

3 ounces asparagus juice
4 medium carrots, juiced
1 radish, juiced

3 ounces spinach juice
4 ounces watercress juice
1 green onion, juiced

Combine all ingredients.

Makes 1 serving

TROPICAL TEMPTATION

1 Hawaiian papaya, peeled
   and seeded
2 Hayden mangoes, peeled
   and seeded

1 pound peeled and cored
   ripe pineapple
2 kiwi, peeled

Place ingredients in a blender and blend for 1 minute, until liquefied.

Makes 3 to 4 servings

MOOLESS MILK

2 cups soaked and peeled   3 cups pure water*
   raw almonds
½ teaspoon nonalcoholic
   vanilla

Place ingredients in a blender. Blend for 2 minutes, until liquefied. Strain contents into a pitcher.

Makes 2 servings

BANANA SHAKE

1½ frozen bananas   1 or 2 drops liquid stevia*
1½ cups pure water*

Place ingredients in a blender. Blend for 1 minute, until liquefied.

Makes 1 serving

THREE GRAIN MILK

1 cup sprouted oats   1 cup sprouted kamut*
1 cup sprouted spelt*   6 cups pure water*

Place ingredients in a blender. Blend for 3 minutes, until liquefied. Strain contents into a pitcher and serve.

Makes 4 to 6 servings

Menus for One Week

Sunday
Breakfast: Purest Green Drink and/or toasted Sprouted Grain Bread
Lunch: Leafy Avocado Salad
             Italian Whole Bread
Dinner: Butternut Smooth Soup
             Asparagus with Shakti Mushrooms
             Fresh Organic Fruit Pie

Monday
Breakfast: Live Vert Juice and/or sprouted teff grain
Lunch: Essene Rye Crisp
             Almost Tuna Salad
Dinner: Basic Seed Soup
             Pine Nut Patty
             Yam Pie

Tuesday

Breakfast: Herbs in a Glass and/or sprouted quinoa
Lunch: Tasty Grainy Stuff
            Stuffed Peppers
Dinner: Barley Soup
            Cauliflower Loaf
            Creamy Apple-Walnut Pudding

Wednesday

Breakfast: Queen's Juice and/or Sprouted Corn Porridge
Lunch: Spanish Cracker
            Corn and Mushroom Salad
Dinner: Autumn Soup
            Sesame Sensation
            Avocado Cups

Thursday

Breakfast: Power Pure Juice and/or sprouted amaranth
Lunch: Multi-Grain Thin Bread
            Broccoli and Cauliflower Salad
Dinner: Vegetable Soup
            Guacamole Dinner
            Old World Carrot Cake

Friday

Breakfast: Italian Stallion and/or toasted Sprouted Grain Bread
Lunch: Tasty Grainy Stuff
            Potato and Squash Salad
Dinner: Autumn Soup
            Wheat Casserole
            Carob Banana Ice-Bar

Saturday

Breakfast:	Living and Loving Juice and/or sprouted buckwheat
Lunch:	Essene Rye Crisp
	Complete Meal Salad
Dinner:	Raw Celery Soup
	Buckwheat Green Stem Pasta
	Flaming Fruit

Epilogue

The twentieth century has been innovative for the food industry. With great speed, the food revolution whisked us along on a high-tech journey that promised government-controlled quality, low prices, fast-food convenience, and abundant supply. Now as we enter the new millennium, we can see that this journey has gone off track; we've ventured down a road that robs us of daily vitality, exuberant health, and longevity. Fortunately, the mass population is giving signs that it is ready to admit the mistake and move in a new direction—toward living-foods vegetarianism.

The success of the living-foods lifestyle has been proven over the last several decades, and testimonials of its ability to restore health and energy to the human body continue to pour into the Hippocrates Health Institute every day. Now, the secret is yours. You have the information, the knowledge, the scientific support, and the step-by-step program offered in this book to jump onto the right track. As you discard poisonous foods and negative attitudes and adopt a living-foods diet, each cell in your body will be charged by the oxygen, enzymes, and billions of electrical cells fueled by this food; this will raise the energy level of every living cell within you and increase your ability to live life to its fullest, most glorious potential.

Notes

Chapter 1

1. Mikkel Hindhede, "The Effect of Food Restrictions During War on Mortality in Copenhagen," *Journal of the American Medical Association* 74,6 (1920): 381.
2. Chen Junshi, T. C. Campbell, Li Junyao, R. Reto, *Diet, Lifestyle and Mortality in China* (Oxford University Press and Cornell University Press, 1990).
3. National Research Council, National Academy of Sciences, *Diet and Health* (Washington, DC: 1989), 57.
4. A. H. Lindsay, E. A. Oddoye, S. Margen, "Protein-Induced Hypercalciuria: A Longer Term Study," *American Journal of Clinical Nutrition* 32 (1979): 741–49.
5. Alberto Ascherio, Eric B. Rimm, Meir J. Stampfer, et al, "Dietary Intake of Marine n-3 Fatty Acids, Fish Intake, and the Risk of

Coronary Disease Among Men," *The New England Journal of Medicine,* 332, 15 (April 13, 1995): 977–82.

6. PrimeTime Live, "Something's Fishy." ABC television network, John Quinones (correspondent), Robert Campos (producer). Feb. 3, 1994.

7. United States Environmental Protection Agency. *National Study of Chemical Residues in Fish Fact Sheet.* Washington, DC: Office of Science and Technology, Nov. 1992, EPA 823-F-92-001.

8. Sandra Jacobson, et al., "The Effect of Intrauterine PCB Exposure on Visual Recognition Memory," *Child Development* 56 (1985): 853–60.

9. Devra L. Davis and H. L. Bradlow. "Suspecting Hormonal Mimicking Chemicals in the Environment Contributes to Many Breast Cancers." *Scientific American,* October 1995.

10. United States Department of Agriculture. *Pesticide Data Program: Progress Report,* June 1995.

Chapter 2

1. E. B. Szekely, *The Essene Science of Life* (Cartago, Costa Rica: International Biogenic Society, 1978).

2. Max Gerson, *A Cancer Therapy: Results of Fifty Cases* (Del Mar, CA: Totality Books, 1977).

3. Paul Kouchakoff, "The Influence of Food Cooking on the Blood Formula of Man," *Proceedings of First International Congress of Microbiology,* Paris, 1930.

4. Edward Howell, *Food Enzymes for Health and Longevity* (Woodstock Valley, CT: Omangod Press, 1946).

5. Edward Howell, *Enzyme Nutrition* (Wayne, NJ: Avery Publishing, 1985).

6. Anthony Sebastian, Steven T. Harris, Joan H. Ottaway, et al, "Improved Mineral Balance and Skeletal Metabolism in Postmenopausal Women Treated with Potassium Bicarbonate," *The New England Journal of Medicine* (June 23, 1994): 1776.

7. B. Gurskin, "Chlorophyll — Its Therapeutic Place in Acute and Supporative Disease," *American Journal of Surgery* 49 (1940): 49–55.

8. Lois M. Miller, "The Green Magic of Chlorophyll," *Reader's Digest* (April, 1941): 30–32.

9. John Gainer, "Now the Villain Is Protein," *Science News* (August 21, 1971): 123–24.

10. Kouchakoff, "The Influence of Food Cooking on the Blood Formula of Man."

11. Otto Warburg, "The Prime Cause and Prevention of Cancer," trans. by Dean Burk. (Bethesda, MD: National Cancer Institute, 1969).

12. *A Diet for All Reasons*. Narrated by Michael Klaper, M.D., 60 minutes, Nutritional Services, 1992, videocassette.

13. Francis Pottenger, *Pottenger's Cats: A Study in Nutrition* (La Mesa, CA: Price-Pottenger Nutrition Foundation, 1983).

Chapter 3

1. Wayne Hearn, "Studies Create Confusion, But Eating Greens Is Good," *American Medical News* (May 9, 1994): 20.

2. Sharon Begley, "Beyond Vitamins," *Newsweek* (April 25, 1994): 45–49.

3. Hector E. Solorzano del Rio, "Systemic Enzyme Therapy," *Townsend Letter for Doctors* (May 1995): 76–86.

4. Milina MacPhee, Kenneth P. Chepenik, Rebecca A. Liddell, Kelly K. Nelson, Linda D. Siracusa, and Arthur M. Buchberg, "The Secretory Phospholipase A2 Gene Is a Candidate for the Mom1 Locus, A Major Modifier of ApcMin-Induced Intestinal Neoplasia," *Cell* 81 (June 16, 1995): 957–66.

5. Beatrice Trum Hunter, "Dietary Recommendations for Certain Health Conditions," *Consumers Research Magazine* (June 1993): 8.

6. Richard Adamson, "Mutagens and Carcinogens in the Diet," *Progress in Clinical and Biological Research* 347 (1990): 323–25.

7. M. G. Knize, P. L. Cunningham, E. A. Griffin, et al, "Characterization of Mutagenic Activity in Cooked-Grain-Food Products," *Food and Chemical Toxicology* 32 (1994).

8. Ann Wigmore, *The Hippocrates Diet and Health Program* (Wayne, NJ: Avery, 1984).

9. Pnina Bar-Sella, "Chlorophyll: The Active Factor in Wheat Sprout Extract Inhibiting the Metabolic Activation of Carcinogens in Vitro," *Nutrition and Cancer* 1, 3 (1995).

10. Arthur B. Robinson, Arnold Hunsberger, Fred C. Westall, "Suppression Of Squamous Cell Carcinoma in Hairless Mice by Dietary Nutrient Variation," *Mechanisms of Aging and Development* 76 (1994): 201–214.

11. Debbie Galant, "Eat, Drink, and Be Healthy," *Rutgers Magazine,* 75, 1 (Spring 1995): 18.

12. Devra L. Davis and H. L. Bradlow, "Can Environmental Estrogens Cause Breast Cancer?" *Scientific American* (October 1995): 168–72.

13. "Diet and Stress and Vascular Disease," *Journal of the American Medical Association* 176, 9 (June 3, 1961): 806.

14. John McDougall, *The McDougall Plan* (New York: New American Library, 1991).

15. John Robbins, *Diet for a New America* (Walpole, NH: Stillpoint Publishing, 1987).

16. P. Lucas, "Dietary Fat Aggravates Active Rheumatoid Arthritis," *Clinical Research,* 29 (1981): 754A.

17. A. Parke, "Rheumatoid Arthritis and Food," *British Medical Journal,* 282 (1981): 2027.

18. Kenneth H. Cooper, *Antioxidant Revolution* (Nashville, TN: Thomas Nelson Publishers, 1994).

Chapter 4

1. O. Carl Simonton, S. Matthews-Simonton, J. Creighton, *Getting Well Again* (New York: Bantam Books, 1981).

2. Julio Licinio, P. W. Gold, M. Wong, "A Molecular Mechanism for Stress-Induced Alterations in Susceptibility to Disease," *The Lancet* 346 (1995): 104–6.
3. B. Klopfer, "Psychological Variables in Human Cancer," *Journal of Projective Techniques and Personality Assessment* 21 (1957): 321–40.
4. R. Glaser, J. K. Kiecolt-Glaser, C. Speicher, et al., "Stress, Loneliness, and Changes in Herpes Virus Latency," *Journal of Behavioral Medicine* 8 (1985): 249–60.
5. J. K. Kiecolt-Glaser, L. Fisher, P. Ogrocki, et al., "Marital Quality, Marital Disruption, and Immune Function," *Psychosomatic Medicine* 49 (1987): 13–34.
6. L. Luborksy, V. J. Brightman, A. H. Katcher, "Herpes Simplex Virus and Moods: A Longitudinal Study," *Journal of Psychosomatic Research* 20 (1976): 543–48.
7. M. Kemeny, F. Cohen, L. Zegans, "Psychological and Immuniological Predictors of Genital Herpes Recurrence," *Psychosomatic Medicine* 51 (1989): 195–208.
8. R. K. Wallace and H. Benson, "The Physiology of Meditation," *Scientific American* 226 (1972): 84–90.

Chapter 5

1. Robert C. Atkins, *Dr. Atkins' Diet Revolution* (New York: David McKay Co., 1972).
2. Irwin M. Stillman and Sam Sinclair Baker, *Dr. Stillman's 14-Day Shape-Up Program* (New York: Delacorte Press, 1974).
3. Herman Tarnower, *The Complete Scarsdale Medical Diet* (New York: Rawson, Wade Publishers, 1978).
4. Ibid.
5. Atkins.
6. Nathan Pritikin, *The Pritikin Program for Diet and Exercise* (New York: Grosset and Dunlap, 1979).
7. Sheldon Margen and Dale A. Ogar, "Fake Fat Warning." *The Record,* Jan. 10, 1996, footnote 4.

Chapter 7

1. Jesse Ross, "Biological Effects of Pulsed High Peak Power Electromagnetic Energy Using Diapulse." *Emerging Electromagnetic Medicine,* Ed. M. E. O'Connor (New York: Springer-Verlag, 1990): 271–78.

Chapter 8

1. T. W. Carlat, *Organically Grown Food: A Consumer's Guide.* (Los Angeles: Wood Publishing, 1990).
2. Ibid.
3. Mary Wolff, "Blood Levels of Organochlorine Residues and Risk of Breast Cancer," *Journal of the National Cancer Institute* 85, 8 (April 21, 1993): 648–52.
4. Department of Agriculture, Agricultural Marketing Service, "Pesticide Data Program: Annual Summary Calendar Year 1993," June 1995.
5. Carlat.
6. Andrea Rock, "Vitamin Hype: Why We're Wasting $1 of Every $3 We Spend," *Money* 24, 9 (September 1995): 83–92.
7. National Cancer Institute, "Beta Carotene and Vitamin A Halted in Lung Cancer Prevention Trial," press release, Jan. 18, 1996.
8. Ibid.

Chapter 9

1. G. H. Erp-Thomas, *A New Concept in Diet* (Boston: Rising Sun Publication, 1978).

Ingredient Glossary

Most of these ingredients can be found in health food stores and Asian markets.

adzuki: small, dark-red beans, renowned for their high-quality protein and health benefits to the renal organs. Also known as azuki or aduki.

agar: a clear, flavorless sea vegetable. It is freeze-dried, sold in sticks or flakes, and used like gelatin.

amaranth: an Aztec grain renowned for its bone-strengthening properties

arame: a thin, black sea vegetable with a mild flavor

Braggs Aminos: a complete liquid protein (not fermented) that is a good substitute for nonorganic salt or soy sauce

dulse: a northern ocean sea vegetable high in minerals

jicama: a sweet-tasting root vegetable

kamut: a primitive form of wheat

kelp: a large, calcium-rich sea vegetable often sold powdered or in capsules

kombu: a thick, protein- and mineral-rich sea vegetable

meal (almond, sesame seed, sunflower seed):   seeds or grains ground without water to create a coffee-grainlike consistency

miso: a salty paste made from cooked, aged soybeans and sometimes grains. Thick and spreadable, it's used for flavoring and soup bases.

nori: a dried sea vegetable sold in sheet, commonly used to make sushi

psyllium: a seed that swells and produces a medicinal gel when moist. Used in recipes, it can help create a healthier intestinal tract.

psyllium powder: psyllium seeds ground up into a more digestible form

pure water: distilled or reverse osmosis water

quinoa: a high-protein South American grain

seed sauce: made by mixing 2 cups ground seeds such as sunflower or pumpkin with 1 cup water

spelt: a primitive form of wheat

stevia: sugar substitute derived from an herb, which is sold in both liquid and powdered form

tamari: a naturally brewed soy sauce that contains no sugar and is available wheat-free

tahini: a thick, smooth paste made from ground sesame seeds

tempeh: a cultured food made from soybeans and sometimes grains

wakame: a nutritious sea vegetable

Index